LIZ EARLE
SKIN

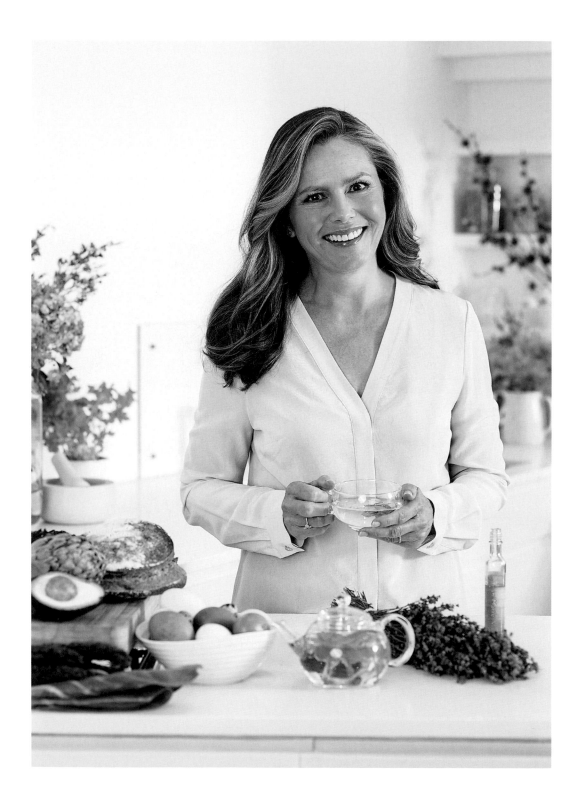

LIZ EARLE

SKIN

DELICIOUS RECIPES &
THE ULTIMATE WELLBEING PLAN FOR
RADIANT SKIN IN 6 WEEKS

For my girls – all of you

First published in Great Britain in 2016
by Orion Spring, an imprint of the Orion Publishing Group Ltd
Carmelite House
50 Victoria Embankment
London, EC4Y 0DZ
An Hachette UK Company
10 9 8 7 6 5 4 3 2

A CIP catalogue record for this book is available from the British Library.
ISBN: 978 1 4091 6414 2

Photographers: Dan Jones and Lorenzo Mazzega
Creative director: Helen Ewing
Home economist and food stylist: Natalie Thomson
Editor: Jinny Johnson
Project editor: Jillian Young
Copy editor: Liz Jones
Nutritional analysis calculated by: Fiona Hunter

Printed in Italy

*Every effort has been made to ensure that the information in this book is accurate.
The information will be relevant to the majority of people but may not be applicable
in each individual case, so it is advised that professional medical advice is obtained
for specific health matters. Neither the publisher nor author accept any legal responsibility
for any personal injury or other damage or loss arising from the use or misuse of the information
in this book. Anyone making a change in their diet should consult their GP, especially if
pregnant, infirm, elderly or under 16.*

www.orionbooks.co.uk

Contents

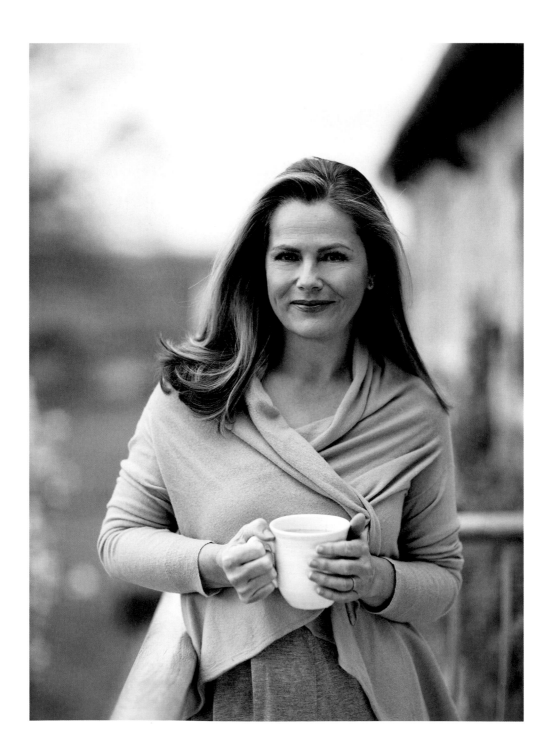

Introduction

Caring for skin has been a lifelong passion. I've spent the last thirty years researching and writing about how to achieve a healthy, more radiant-looking complexion. In studying the skin, I've been fortunate to work with world class academics and leading researchers to discern the very best skincare advice. This has led me to create the fool-proof plan in this book to literally eat your way to better skin.

SKIN is all about how to create smoother, clearer, softer and younger-looking skin at any age (I'm in my fifties and firmly believe it's never too late to see a visible difference). Part One of the book is my six-week plan, with each week focussing on a different aspect of skincare – from detox and exfoliation, cleansing and healing, to nourishing, balance and, finally, radiance and maintenance. With this six-week skin plan also comes the added benefits of better health, improved energy levels, sounder sleep and an overall boost to your wellbeing.

Part Two has 70 delicious and easy recipes to accompany the six-week plan in Part One, but they are sure to be enjoyed when you aren't following the plan, too. This surely is the most enjoyable way to eat yourself beautiful!

Our skin is a powerful outward expression of what's happening inside. So a healthy outer glow is dependent on a healthy internal body. It really is a win-win. Feeding our faces also feeds every single cell in our body, from brain cells to muscle fibres, with a positive boost to our immune system along the way. Visible skin disorders may be a manifestation that all is not well beneath the surface, so as well as helping to create a gorgeously healthy glow, this simple six-week plan is also likely to leave you feeling so much better too. I've also included advice for sorting out troublesome skin issues, from early adolescent breakouts to menopausal wrinkles, as well as dietary and practical skincare tips to help with eczema, psoriasis, rosacea and much more.

As you will read in this book, I'm passionate about dispelling beauty myths and sorting out fact from fiction, no easy task given the obfuscation and confusion amidst a mass of online information. Creating a range of skincare with worldwide acclaim for Liz Earle Beauty Co. certainly helped to give me an insight into the realities of product formulation – and a genuine knowledge of what does (and doesn't) work.

I have a deep love and respect for natural ingredients, including plant oils and botanicals, and especially love to use many of these fabulous skin savers in recipes in this book. From seed oils such as evening primrose oil (Rigel seed is the most effective kind) to high-altitude lavender (it has the best scent), nature has so many wonderful skin-caring ingredients that are also renewable and sustainable for our planet. From the A-Z of argan oil to za'atar herbs, I'm a big fan of potent plants.

So it may come as something of a surprise to read that I also advocate turning to conventional medicine to treat acute adolescent acne (in my view, absolutely essential to prevent permanent skin scarring) and to hear that after many years of in-depth study, I agree with the consensus of researchers who say that the parabens used in skincare are not only safe, but desirable (see page 15 for more information on this).

If I have learnt one thing over the decades, it is that there is always more to learn. My research has taken me all over the world, from the hallowed halls of Harvard Medical School to indigenous tribeswomen in Kenya, Uganda and Malawi. From cutting-edge academia to ancient folklore, I've distilled the very essence of what our skin really needs to radiate with the glow of good health. You'll find much of what I've learnt on these pages, as well as further resources for personal follow-up and supplier information at the back of this book (see page 247). You won't find many specific beauty product references on these pages though, as I believe it's up to you to take the principles of what I'm about to share and apply it to your own lifestyle, budget and personal preference. I think it's important for you to feel empowered to personalise your own regime – and not be dictated to with a prescriptive rigidity that is all too common in the beauty industry.

As well as looking at what we put onto our skin, so much of what makes us look and feel beautiful comes from what we put into our bodies, in the form of food and drink, as well as the way we live. My focus has always been on making feel-good-food that the whole family will love to eat, as well as creating successful eating strategies to give us the glow of great skin. I have five children, two in their twenties, two in their teens and a tiny tot for good measure – so I make all my recipes with a broad range of ages in mind. You can be sure that these amazing recipes, from breakfasts to brunch, lunch, skin snacks right through to supper dishes and more, have been tested and approved by my very own informal tasting committee. If we don't all love a recipe, I change it and tweak it to make it just perfect.

The second part of this book is all about eating for better skin and I encourage low-carb, low-sugar, high-quality protein meals, with lots of healthy skin-saving fats and oils, probiotics and some supplements, as well as lots of fresh vegetables (mostly green) and certain fruits (such as anthocyanin-rich berries) too. Accessible and easy to make, many of my recipes in this book are time-tested favourites I turn to time and time again at home.

In my recipes I have provided nutritional advice including calorie counts per serving and dietary guidance as shown by:

V VEGETARIAN

DF DAIRY-FREE

GF GLUTEN-FREE

These guides do not include ingredients or sides offerered as serving suggestions or tips, so keep this in mind if you are watching your calorie intake or if you have allergy intolerances.

I hope you love following my six-week plan to radiance. I'd love to hear how you get on so do please share your success stories along the way using #skinfood to show and inspire others that fabulous skin is truly achievable at any age – you'll find my details on page 256.

With love,

Liz x

lizearlewellbeing.com

PART ONE:
SIX-WEEK PLAN

WEEK ONE:
Detox and Exfoliation

Start your plan with a big clear-out. Help rid not only your cupboards but also your body of unwanted substances that hinder the skin – and make a fresh start. Stock-up on the more internally cleansing ingredients, such as green leafy veggies, fresh ginger root and plain live yoghurt. Invest in a water filter jug if you don't already have one and be prepared to enjoy some new foods.

This week you may like to get your day off to a skin-saving start with my Cinnamon-toasted Oats with Yoghurt and Summer Fruit (page 92). Swapping out the more usual pasta and potato carbs for a skin-friendly low-GL (glycaemic load – see page 45) lentil dish is also a good option. My Lentils with Rainbow Vegetables and Kale Pesto (page 178) are simply sensational!

① Inside: Detox your fridge and food cupboards, and make smart swaps

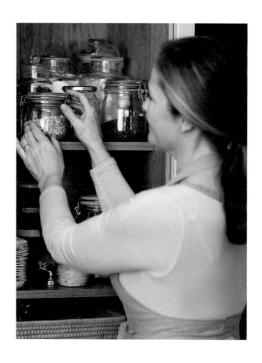

Our skin mirrors the condition of our body on the inside. All the great creams and potions in the world won't make you truly radiant if your diet isn't also skin friendly, so looking at what we eat is the first step in our six weeks to great skin.

Most of us know how to eat healthily – there is so much good advice around nowadays – but it's all too easy to let bad habits build up. Many processed foods, for example, contain too much sugar and salt, as well as synthetic colourings and other unhelpful additives. We're not likely to take in enough of these to do us serious harm, but it's not hard to see how our bodies can get overloaded – and this can show up on our faces as dull, dingy skin.

It's good to go right back to basics, cutting out processed foods as far as possible and eating fresh food that's had as little done to it as possible. Even apparently healthy fruit and veg may be coated with pesticides and fungicides, so give them a good scrub in soapy water and rinse and dry well before using. Consider buying organic produce if you can – farm box delivery schemes are handy, and usually good value.

Start your 'detox' week by clearing out your fridge and food cupboards. If biscuits, cakes and processed stuff aren't readily to hand, you're not going to be so tempted. Instead, make sure you're well stocked with fresh, nourishing foods, such as whole grains (short-grain brown rice is one of my favourites), seasonal vegetables and fruit, as well as nuts and seeds and other healthy snacks. I certainly don't want to encourage waste, but this is also a good time to get rid of any stale herbs and spices that won't do your cooking or your body any favours, as well as those long-forgotten, almost empty jars at the back of the fridge. Chuck out anything that doesn't smell right. Check dates on foods such as pulses and nuts (they can go stale and rancid, especially if they get too warm) and make sure you move those that need using soonest to the front of the shelf.

Audit your freezer, too, and check packaging and labels. Cook anything that needs using up, and compost foods that are spoiled.

SMART SWAPS

- Finish up any cereal, and re-stock with porridge oats instead. Consider making your own muesli (see page 94), which is likely to be much healthier than anything you can buy ready-made.

- Stop buying flavoured yoghurts and go for live natural yoghurt instead. You can also try to make your own (see page 92).

- Cut out the crisps. If you fancy something crispy without the calories, try thinly slicing a bagel and baking until crisp. These make good low-fat crispy bites (or use them for dips). Stock up with nuts as well as sunflower and pumpkin seeds. Try making some of my beauty bombs to snack on (see pages 132–135).

- Fill your shelves with lentils and other pulses, dried or in cans. Make sure you have stocks of the more unusual healthy grains such as quinoa and freekeh, both great for quick, sustaining, skin-friendly meals.

- Try spelt flour instead of plain white, and go for spelt or buckwheat pasta or noodles. They provide slow-release energy instead of insulin-surging sugar spikes.

- Avoid shop-bought dressings and sauces and go for good natural oils, such as olive, nut and avocado – all great for the skin, and some of my favourite internal skin-plumpers.

② Outside: Detox bathroom cupboards and your make-up bag, too

This is a good moment to have a long hard look at your bathroom cupboards and make-up stocks. It's not a good idea to overload our skin with lots of different products, so find what suits you and stick to it. I've used the same three-step Cleanse, Tone and Moisturise regime for over 20 years.

Inevitably, our shelves tend to get filled with impulse buys, samples and unwanted gifts, so have a good sort out. Give away anything you don't like or will never use. Check use-by dates and throw away any products that smell bad. Most products have an open-lid icon with 6M, 12M or 18M printed on the base, indicating how many months these can be kept after opening. Wash your make-up brushes and bags using shampoo.

Mascara and lipsticks can harbour bacteria from our eyes and mouths so, strictly speaking, should only be kept for three or four months (and never shared), then thrown away. Prolong the life of your mascara by making sure you screw the wand in properly – if air gets into the mascara it deteriorates faster. Don't keep them for longer than six months or so – it's easy to get eye and eyelid infections from contaminated cosmetics, which is why preservatives in these are so essential.

When choosing products, I prefer to look for those containing natural plant-based ingredients and plant oils. Check labels carefully and avoid anything with sodium lauryl/laureth sulphate (SLS), particularly for use on your face. Studies have shown that this chemical can irritate the skin, especially if you're dry-skinned or prone to eczema.

READING LABELS

It's worth learning how to read labels – a small magnifying glass is useful as the print is often so tiny. Cosmetic and toiletry labels must, by law, include an ingredient listing. This is called the International Nomenclature of Cosmetic Ingredients (INCI). This is a system for standardising names of ingredients such as waxes, oils, pigments, preservatives and so on based on their scientific names (often in Latin), so they can be read worldwide. For example, water is listed as *Aqua*. Each ingredient is listed in order of quantity, so *Aqua* is likely to appear first, followed by an ingredient such as shea butter (*Butyrospermum parkii*). Smaller amounts of ingredients appear towards the end, such as vitamin E (*Tocopherol*), fragrances (*Parfum*) and preservatives (such as phenoxyethanol).

Learning how to read a label can make us especially savvy when it comes to buying skincare: a product may proudly declare itself to be full of shea butter, but if on closer inspection you see it appearing towards the end of the list, then you can be fairly sure it's more myth and marketing than beauty beneficial. Don't be shy of preservatives. They are essential for keeping products safe, and much that has been written about them has been shown to be scaremongering and wrong.

PARABENS

One of the biggest skincare scare stories in recent years has surrounded the use of a group of preservatives called parabens. They were first linked to breast cancer in 2004, in a single PhD study considered seriously flawed by many experts. This one study, poorly interpreted, created a media-fuelled consumer panic, leading to almost all skincare manufacturers feeling compelled to remove parabens from products. In an interview for this book, the author of the original study personally admitted that there is no conclusive link between parabens and breast cancer. In addition, numerous international studies continue to show parabens to be a safe and effective form of preserving skincare. The undisputed truth is that parabens occur naturally in everyday fruits and vegetables (apples last longer than strawberries as they contain more parabens) and the aromatic organic acid 4-hydroxybenzoic acid (which forms the basis of parabens) is the most commonly occurring organic acid in the vegetable kingdom. It's an essential part of plant life – and therefore our diet. When used in skincare, the family of parabens preservatives are also amongst the least likely to cause a sensitive skin reaction, unlike many of their replacements.

③ Inside: Sugar – cut it down, cut it out

In the form of sweet foods and white refined carbs, sugar is the enemy of dieters; we all know it piles on the pounds. Research also suggests that sugar is at the root of much ill-health – and it is bad for your skin. If you have a high-sugar diet your skin will suffer like the rest of your body.

This is the result of a process known as glycation. When we have large amounts of sugar in the body, the sugar molecules attach themselves to protein molecules and form advanced glycation end products (AGEs). The more sugar in your body, the more AGEs will be formed. For our skin this is bad news. Skin proteins collagen and elastin are particularly susceptible to AGEs, so if your diet is high in sugar your skin is likely to wrinkle and age more quickly. You will also be more prone to inflammatory skin conditions, such as acne and rosacea.

When you look at your diet with a view to cutting down on sugar, it's important to remember that it is not just cakes and the spoonfuls in your tea you need to watch for, it's also refined carbohydrates such as white bread, white rice and pasta. Once digested these become sugar in the body. Fruit is high in sugar, but nature packages it with fibre and plenty of other good things, like vitamin C and beta-carotene, which are good for the skin.

Cutting out sugar in your tea and coffee and avoiding those biscuits, sweets and white bread might be hard, but at least it's straightforward. What's trickier is avoiding the hidden sugar in foods that you wouldn't normally expect, such as tomato ketchup, canned soups, sauces and ready meals. Check labels for sugar content and avoid processed foods. Look at where sugar comes in the ingredients list – the higher up it is, the greater the quantity.

You can use artificial sweeteners, but some medics have concerns about their safety, and they don't help to re-educate your taste buds to enjoy less-sweet foods. I prefer to stick mostly to fruit, dried fruit and small amounts of plant syrup and honey, with only the occasional spoonful of sugar. I also use dark chocolate as a sweet treat, and the great news is that small amounts are actually good for you! Stick with at least 70 per cent cocoa solids, which is rich in natural antioxidants and minerals. The high cocoa content has been shown to increase blood circulation to the upper layers of the skin, helping to give us a healthy glow. Don't overdo it though – a couple of squares are enough …

SMART SWAPS

- Swap sugary breakfast cereal for porridge with a sprinkling of naturally sweet, crunchy sunflower seeds or flaked almonds.

- Swap white bread for wholemeal, or try my fabulously easy and delicious Rough and Tumble Bread (see page 231).

- Swap biscuits for oatcakes spread with nut butter (see page 121).

- Swap milk chocolate for a couple of squares of the dark stuff; look for at least 70 per cent cocoa solids on the label.

④ Outside: Start dry-skin body brushing

Body brushing is an easy, inexpensive treat for your skin and a great way to kick-start the day. You can do it yourself at home – all you need is a brush and a few moments of your time. It feels odd at first, but trust me on this one – once you get into the habit, you'll love it, I promise.

Our skin is constantly eliminating waste products, and dry-skin brushing helps to remove these. It also boosts our circulation, exfoliates the skin naturally and smooths out little lumps and bumps

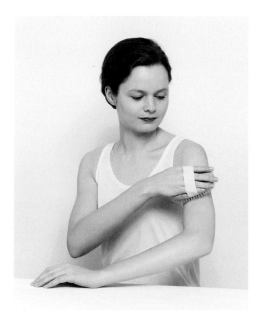
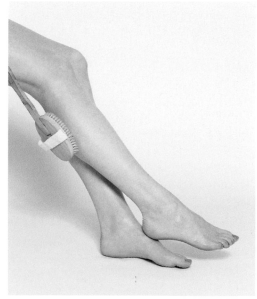

– it's really great for improving the appearance of cellulite. Brushing is best done in the morning before you step into the shower – if you stand in the light you'll see scores of tiny skin cells hit the air. Choose a good natural bristle brush that's firm enough to create friction but not so hard as to scratch or hurt your skin. The brush should have a good long handle to make it easier for you to reach all parts of your body, and it should always be used dry, on dry skin.

Start by brushing the soles of your feet, then work up your legs to your thighs and buttocks, using slow, upward strokes. Go gently over your stomach but don't brush your breasts (the skin there is too fragile). Brush up your arms from your wrists to your shoulders – brushing is especially good for improving bumpy, pimply skin on flabby upper arms. Brush across your shoulders and down your back. Try to always brush towards your heart, as this helps the flow of lymph in the body. Avoid brushing any very sensitive areas or broken skin.

When you're done, shower and moisturise as usual. You'll soon notice the difference in your skin. Keep your brush just for you and wash it carefully every week, leaving it to air-dry naturally.

⑤ Inside: Cut caffeine and alcohol

Caffeine is a diuretic, so it dehydrates the body – not good news for the skin. It also increases the load on our liver, meaning that toxins (unwanted waste material the body naturally processes) are more likely to build up and manifest as skin problems.

I love my coffee, so I sometimes find my intake is creeping up and I have to cut back. I find total withdrawal just too sudden, as I get caffeine-withdrawal headaches, so I cut down on coffee and strong tea by one cup a day, until I'm down to one small mug a day at breakfast. From there, it's easier to cut caffeine out altogether if you want to.

Start the day with a mug of hot water with a spritz of lemon instead. This gets the liver working and is a great way to reboot your metabolism after a night's sleep. Lemon juice is detoxifying, cleansing and energising and packed with skin-friendly vitamin C. The rest of the day I tend to drink cleansing herb and spice teas, which are refreshing and do the skin lots of good. Fresh mint is an excellent internal cleanser and all you have to do is to steep a bunch of mint leaves in hot water for a few minutes, then strain; perfect after meals as a digestion aid and stomach soother. Nettle and fennel teas are also excellent and are available as dried loose teas and tea bags. Both are recommended frequently by herbalists as cleansing tonics, and are rich in antioxidants, vitamins and minerals.

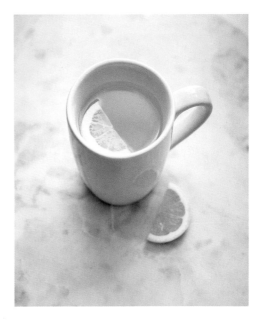

Another drink I enjoy instead of coffee or tea is a spicy infusion of a few slices of fresh root ginger steeped in hot water (you can add a little honey, too). It's antibacterial and an excellent system cleanser. Ginger is also known to be good for nausea or sickness – and hangovers!

That brings me to alcohol. Again, this can swiftly overload the liver and dehydrate the skin. Heavy drinkers may also find they get broken veins on the nose and cheeks. I must admit to liking a glass of wine, but it's a good plan to cut your intake right down during this six-week plan to give your liver a break. You'll see the difference in your skin. I find dark spirits and white wine are the worst offenders, so if you do want a little something, content yourself with the very occasional glass of good red wine – preferably organic – or a single shot of good-quality vodka with freshly squeezed fruit juice.

Make sure you're drinking plenty of water (at least 1.6 litres), preferably filtered to remove the chlorine and nitrates, every day. It has tremendous benefits for your health and your skin.

⑥ Outside: Make your own face and body scrubs

Our skin is constantly renewing itself, as skin cells die off to be replaced by new ones. Every day we shed countless thousands of dead skin cells, while new plump skin cells are formed beneath the skin's surface. Dead skin cells can clog the pores and lead to skin looking dull and tired, so a gentle scrub in addition to your regular cleansing routine can really help to instantly freshen the complexion. Young skins can take two or more gentle scrubs a week, but those with more mature skin are better off sticking to one.

And don't forget the rest of you. A body scrub is really invigorating and improves the circulation, while leaving skin soft and smooth.

There are plenty of scrubs on the market, but you can make your own very quickly with ingredients from your fridge and store cupboard.

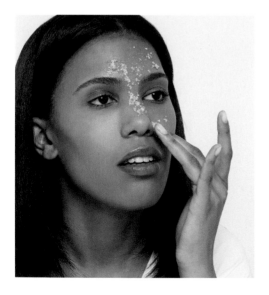
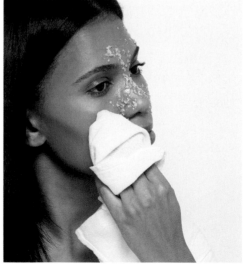

Fabulous Face Scrub

This mixture makes a great weekly treatment to brighten all skin types. The oatmeal helps to soothe the skin, the sugar buffs dead skin cells and the honey has a mildly antibacterial effect. Try to use natural rose water made with real rose oil and not just a synthetic fragrance (it should say 'made with real rose oil' on the label).

15ml (1 tbsp) medium-ground oatmeal
30ml (2 tbsp) rose water (from a pharmacy
  or herbal supplier)

10ml (2 tsp) caster sugar
5ml (1 tsp) runny honey

Mix all the ingredients together in a bowl until they form a gritty paste. Apply to clean skin using gentle circular movements with the fingertips.

Focus on gently scrubbing around the nostrils, chin and forehead to dislodge dead skin cells and unclog the pores. Skin cells are microscopic, so only the smallest amount of pressure is needed to dislodge flakes of dry, dingy skin.

Rinse the skin clean with warm water, and gently pat dry.

Brilliant Body Scrub

This is a brilliant body scrub, as polenta or cornmeal has a good, gritty texture that buffs the body without being too scratchy. It's ideal for pimply areas of skin with poor circulation, such as the thighs or the backs of the upper arms, and is best used once or twice a week on dry or dampened skin, just before stepping into the shower.

30ml (2 tbsp) almond or grapeseed oil
5 drops lavender essential oil

2 drops neroli or petitgrain essential oil
75g polenta or cornmeal

Simply mix the ingredients together to form a gritty paste. The essential oils add a delicious aroma, but you can easily use the scrub without them – it just won't smell as nice – or substitute with your own favourite fragranced oils.

For greater effect, apply with a flannel or soft massage mitt instead of your hands, and massage for 1–2 minutes before rinsing away. This scrub keeps well for a few weeks stored in a screw-top or Kilner jar.

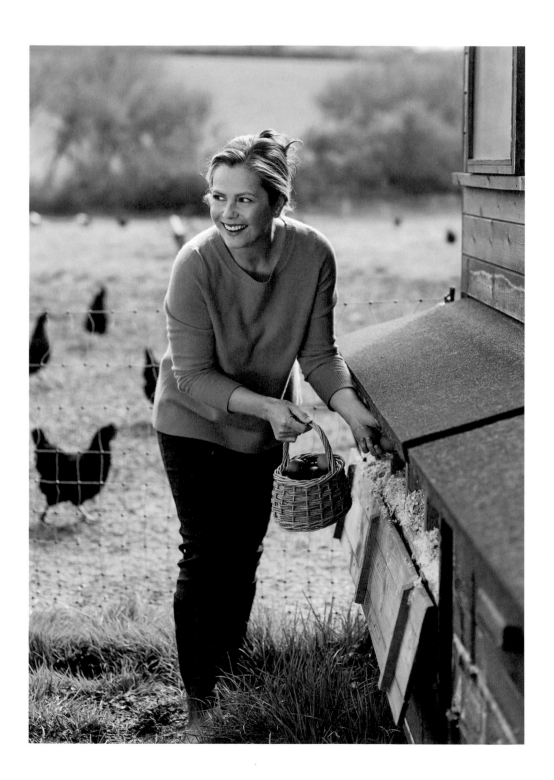

⑦ Inside: Try a two-day inner cleanse

A 48-hour detox is the perfect way to kick-start your programme. The word 'detox' is often derided by the conventional medical establishment, but I take it to mean the ridding of bad habits, giving the body a break from less healthy foods and ways of eating (and drinking), as well as helping to clear the mind, renew energy levels and encourage glowing skin. It's also a good time to rest and aim for better quality sleep – if possible taking a break from phones and other gadgets to reduce stress (or at least just check them occasionally). Do make sure you drink lots of filtered water throughout the day, too. You've already cleared the cupboards and stocked up on healthy foods, so here's what to do.

DAY ONE

Start the day by drinking a glass of hot water with a squeeze of lemon – a great liver cleanser. Do 10 minutes of simple stretches, such as reaching for your toes, then a few minutes of deep peaceful breathing.

Before showering, make sure you spend a few moments body brushing. Treat your body to a skin scrub in the shower, too.

MID-MORNING SNACK

Have a large glass of filtered water and one piece of low-carb fruit, such as an apple, pear or kiwi fruit. Sit down and eat the fruit slowly and mindfully, chewing each mouthful 20 times.

If you can, get out for a walk in the fresh air. Walk briskly and enjoy your surroundings, lifting your head high, neck relaxed and keeping your shoulders down.

LUNCH

Enjoy a simple vegetable broth made with clear stock or vegetable bouillon powder and chopped onions, leeks, carrots, red peppers and celery. Season with freshly ground black pepper and serve with fresh parsley, mint, coriander or a grating of fresh root ginger. Sit down to eat your soup and savour every mouthful.

Rest in the afternoon. Lose yourself in a good book or listen to some music. Sip a big glass of filtered water. After your rest, do some stretches to release any tension in your shoulders and neck. If you're feeling hungry, snack on some carrot, celery or red peppers.

SUPPER

Make yourself a light supper, such as boiled egg or a bowl of high-protein quinoa with plenty of freshly chopped parsley and a good squeeze of lemon. Drink something fresh and herbal such as mint tea.

Run a bath and add a few drops of your favourite essential oil (lavender is very calming). Light some candles, lie back and relax in the peace and quiet. Go to bed early and luxuriate in the bliss of a good night's sleep.

DAY TWO

You should already be feeling invigorated and refreshed, so you might be ready to do a little more than on day one. If you're feeling headachy from lack of caffeine, try to resist but if you have to, drink just one small cup of black tea or coffee.

As on day one, start the day with a glass of hot water with a squeeze of lemon. Do 10 minutes of simple stretches, then enjoy a few minutes of deep peaceful breathing. Before showering, make sure you spend a few moments body brushing.

MID-MORNING SNACK

Choose a piece of low-carb fruit and eat it slowly, as on day one. If your hunger pangs are getting too much, have half a dozen fresh almonds (skin on), chewing them slowly and savouring every mouthful. Have a large glass of filtered water.

Get out for a good walk and make sure you take plenty of deep breaths. Enjoy looking around you and appreciating your surroundings as before.

LUNCH

Make a quick soup with veggies such as carrots, parsnips, leeks, broccoli and cabbage, thickened with some boiled potato and sprinkled with fresh herbs. Eat it slowly and really appreciate the flavours.

Rest with a good book and let yourself drift off for a nap if you like. Do some stretches, yoga or Pilates. Treat yourself to some sticks of raw veg, chewing them well. Drink more water and enjoy feeling so virtuous!

SUPPER

Prepare a small bowl of short-grain brown rice, cooked in filtered water with finely chopped onion. Garnish it with freshly chopped parsley and some sunflower seeds. Chew each mouthful 20 times. Follow with a fresh herb tisane such as camomile or vervain, both soothing and excellent for the digestion.

Give yourself a massage, using almond or grapeseed oil with a few drops of soothing lavender oil. Start with your feet and work up to your neck and shoulders. When you've cleansed your face, apply a facial oil and leave it on overnight to work its magic on your skin. Have another early night and a sound sleep to wake up feeling refreshed and wonderful, ready to face the world again.

Congratulations! You've made a brilliant start and are well on the way to smoother, clearer, more radiant-looking skin!

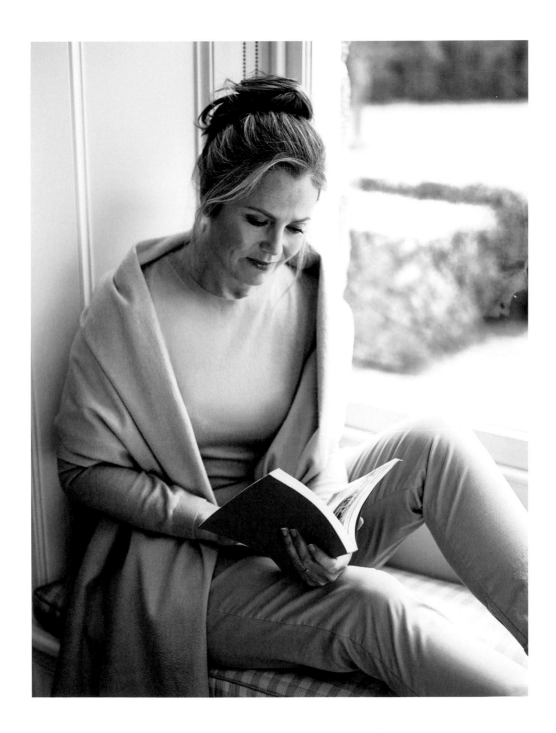

WEEK TWO:
Cleansing

Now you are beautifully 'cleansed' and you've started your routine of body brushing and scrubs, let's concentrate on cleansing. Make sure you're doing everything you can to keep your body clean and fresh – inside and out.

Raising the water-content of our foods is helpful, so I've included plenty of skin-hydrating recipes, such as my ultimate Beauty Broth (page 159). Lettuce Wraps (page (166) are also a perfectly water-rich light bite, along with White Bean, Watercress, Fennel and Tuna Salad (page 138) – truly one of my all-time favourite lunch dishes.

① Outside: Step up your facial cleansing

A thorough cleansing routine is the cornerstone to great skin. My advice is never to use soap or foamy cleansers on the face. They strip our skin of its natural oils and disrupt the pH balance (even 'mild' soaps and cleansing gels can do this). Creamy oil-based cleansers are by far the best for cleaning your skin and for removing make-up.

Look for products containing plant oils, rather than mineral oils. While mineral oils sit on the surface of the skin, plant oils are more easily absorbed into the upper levels of the epidermis and are packed with extra skin-saving nutrients, such as vitamin E. What's more, plant oils are a renewable resource, unlike mineral oils that have to be extracted from the earth (they are a petroleum by-product) and are non-renewable, so not very environmentally friendly.

MORNING

If you've cleaned your face thoroughly before going to bed, you might think a morning cleanse is unnecessary, but in fact it is vital for healthy-looking skin. At night, our skin is busy renewing itself and processing waste matter, which is transferred to dead surface skin cells, so in the morning there are grubby cells to remove as well as the sebum produced overnight, all of which clogs our pores.

Cleanse: Use a creamy cleanser, dotting it on your forehead, cheeks, chin and neck. Massage in well, using small circular movements. Work down your neck, then up from your jawline to your forehead, then out from the centre of your face. Be sure to work around your nostrils. Remove with a pure cotton cloth or thin flannel wrung out in warm water – the cloth has an additional exfoliating effect. Then refresh your skin with the cloth wrung out in cold water.

Tone: Sprinkle an alcohol-free toner on to a cotton-wool pad and smooth it over your face and neck. Work upwards from the jawline and out to the sides of the face. Blot any excess toner with a tissue.

Moisturise: Make sure your hands are clean before dipping a finger into your jar of moisturiser – you don't want to introduce bacteria. Alternatively, use a cotton bud or a small plastic spatula to collect a blob of moisturiser. Dot it over your face and neck and massage in well. Take your moisturiser down the neck and across your upper chest to keep the skin here looking youthful for longer. If you have oily skin, use a lightweight moisturiser and apply only a scant amount over your forehead, nose and chin, with a little more on the cheeks and neck, which are naturally drier areas of skin.

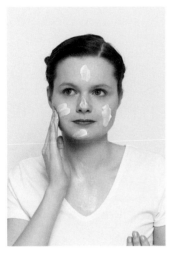 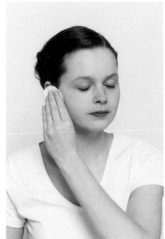 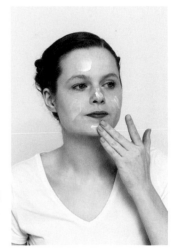

NIGHT

Repeat the morning routine. If you've been wearing foundation you might want to double-cleanse, first to remove the make-up, and then to make sure your skin is really clean.

Tone as before and then moisturise. If you have extra-dry skin, or it's looking a bit devitalised, then apply a few drops of your favourite facial oil to nourish the skin overnight.

If a moisturiser is plant-oil based (that is, it contains no mineral oil), I advocate using a facial oil on top of this. But if your moisturiser contains any form of mineral oil or silicone (such as dimethicone), this creates a barrier on the skin that other ingredients cannot get through. In this case, it is best to apply your facial oil first, then top with the more occlusive moisturiser.

② Inside: Drink more water

Our bodies need water in order to function properly. And, in fact, water makes up two-thirds of our weight and 75 per cent of our brain. Current advice recommends that women drink about eight 200ml glasses of fluid a day – that's about 1.6 litres – and men about ten 200ml glasses – about 2 litres. My own rule is to sip water throughout the day, mostly between meals so as not to dilute the gastric juices required for digestion.

Staying hydrated helps with concentration and relieves fatigue and headaches. If our fluid levels are low it can affect our energy and mood. Drinking plenty also helps us fight infections by flushing toxins from the body faster, and supports heart health. When we are dehydrated the blood gets thicker, so the heart has to pump a little harder.

Staying hydrated also helps with weight control. Often when I think I'm feeling hungry I find a glass of water does the trick – I've actually been in need of fluid, not food.

Although some say that any type of liquid counts towards the total, as do water-rich foods, such as lettuce and cucumber, drinking water is the easiest and healthiest way to quench thirst. My own experience is that I feel and look much better when I drink plenty of pure still water. At home, I drink filtered water from a simple jug filter, but I do occasionally buy bottled water when I'm out and if I've forgotten my re-fillable water bottle.

Most soft drinks, coffees and teas contain additives that are of little benefit to our skin or health. Also, caffeine stimulates the kidneys to produce more urine, which can lead to mild dehydration. Avoid fizzy drinks that contain sugar and colouring – even the diet versions contain synthetic chemicals, colourings and phosphates that are no good for us.

Check your wee
The easiest way to check your hydration levels is to inspect your wee. Generally, it should be light yellow. The darker the colour, the more concentrated it is and the less hydrated you are. Note, though, that your urine will be darker first thing in the morning after a night's sleep. Also, some foods affect the colour of our wee – beetroot, for instance, can give urine a slightly scary pink tinge.

If you do get bored with plain water, there are plenty of ways to make your drinks more appealing.

- Add freshly squeezed lemon or lime juice, cordial or fruit juice to your water.

- At home, keep a big jug of water in the fridge and add flavourings such as slices of cucumber or sprigs of mint and fennel. So refreshing!

- Home-made tisanes and herbal teas are great, especially in the winter when you want a hot drink. Try adding fresh root ginger to hot water, or a stick of cinnamon with a clove. Or make teas with herbs such as peppermint, camomile and fennel.

For more ideas, see the recipes on pages 243–244.

Plastic mountain

Staying hydrated often means carrying a bottle of water with you, but plastic bottles of water have a huge environmental impact. Fossil fuels are used in their manufacture, transportation and refrigeration, and the bottles themselves are a big problem to dispose of. Despite rumours to the contrary, the International Agency for Research on Cancer has found that it is *not* dangerous to reuse plastic bottles, even if they have been kept in the sun: this is a myth that circulates on the Internet. So if you do buy water packed in plastic water bottles, always rinse well and re-use by refilling with filtered tap water for as long as possible. And when you have finished with them, be sure to always put them in the right recycling bin or find alternative uses for them, such as cloches for growing seedlings or freezer containers.

There have also been concerns about the more rigid plastic bottles intended for multiple use that contain a material called Bisphenol A or BPA, which has been linked with reproductive damage and even, potentially, cancer. You can now buy BPA-free bottles and also portable water filter bottles, ideal for carrying around with you. I've listed some of my favourites in the Resources and Suppliers section on page 248.

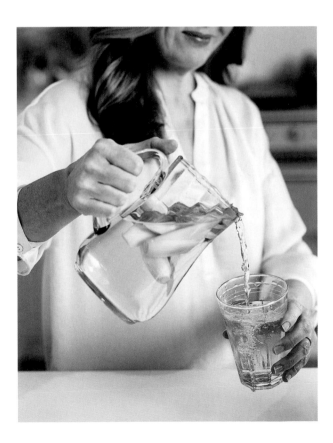

③ Outside: A clean body

Skincare doesn't stop at the neck. It's worth lavishing a little extra care on the rest of our body as well to make sure our skin is radiant and glowing from top to toe. When choosing cleansers for your body, check labels carefully and avoid anything containing sodium lauryl/laureth sulphate (SLS). This ingredient makes a product foam and disrupts the delicate pH balance of the skin, leaving it feeling stripped and sometimes even quite sore. Dermatological studies have shown that SLS-based products can actually trigger eczema in babies and small children, and they are certainly irritants for anyone suffering from the condition.

Instead, look for products containing gentler cleansers such as decyl/coco glucoside, which are extracted from botanicals such as corn and coconut. Soapbark or soapwort are naturally foaming botanicals that are also sometimes used in the more plant-based products. After your shower or bath and while skin is still warm, apply lots of nourishing body cream. I look for those containing plant-based ingredients such as shea butter or cocoa butter (not mineral oil). Be lavish in your application – it really does make a difference.

Back

It's hard to reach your own back, and some of us are prone to spots in this area. Body brushing is great (see pages 16–17) and you can also use a natural fibre back strap with some gentle body wash in the shower to clean your back. The easiest way of moisturising your back is to use a body spray, preferably one containing pure plant oils. For a special treat, ask your partner or a friend to massage you with rich body cream. Or once in a while, you might ask for help to apply a deep-cleansing face mask on your back while you lie on your tummy and relax for 10 minutes.

Breasts

The skin on your neck, décolletage and breasts is fine and extra-sensitive, so needs special care. Don't use a body brush on these areas, but you can apply a gentle facial exfoliator in the shower to keep the skin smooth and free of blemishes. When moisturising your face, always take the moisturiser down on to your chest to keep your cleavage beautifully smooth.

Inevitably, as we get older, gain or lose weight or have children, breasts lose their youthful perkiness, but one way to keep them in good shape is to massage them with nourishing oils. Try adding two drops of essential oil such as fennel, carrot seed or lemongrass to a dessertspoonful of almond or grapeseed oil. Massage around each breast, working towards the armpit using an upward movement, and be sure to include the bra line area. A few minutes once a day is all you need, and it's the perfect way of keeping a health check for any changes to the skin, or for any lumps, bumps or changes in shape or sensitivity.

Elbows and knees

Don't forget to give these often-neglected areas some special attention. After being kept under wraps all winter, elbows and knees can look especially dry and discoloured. A quick and easy remedy is to rub them with a little sugar inside a leftover lemon half to brighten the skin.

④ Inside: Give your liver a break

The liver is the largest of our internal organs and plays a hugely important role in our health. One of its most important tasks is to get rid of waste matter and harmful toxicity in the body – it's the ultimate 'detox' organ. Alcohol, rich food and synthetic chemicals can all put the liver under strain, and you may notice symptoms such as mild headaches, nausea and queasiness – such symptoms used to be described as 'feeling liverish'. Give your liver a much-needed boost by using some liver-supporting herbs. These time-tested bitter-tasting plants stimulate the production of digestive juices and make excellent natural liver cleansers.

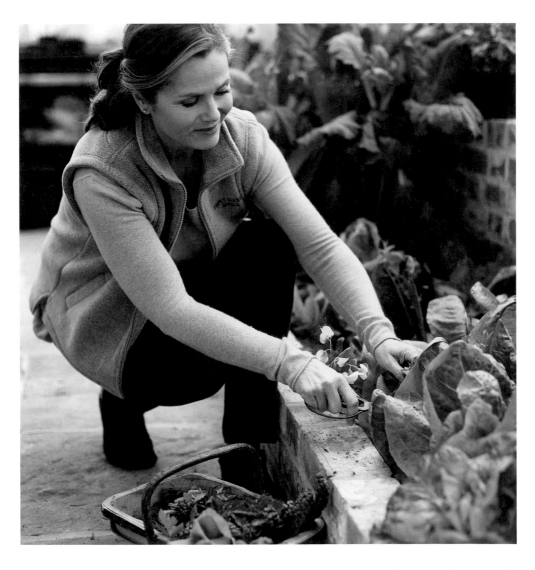

Artichoke

You can eat globe artichokes (see page 33) but artichoke extract, made from the leaves, stems and roots of the plant, is also a good natural liver support. Artichokes belong to the thistle family *Asteraceae* (see Milk thistle, below) and are rich in antioxidant compounds silymarin, caffeic acid and ferulic acid, which can help to protect against damaging free-radical activity. They're also a good source of vitamins C and K, folic acid, copper and iron, as well as being internally cleansing.

Asparagus

Belonging to the same botanical family as onions and garlic, asparagus spears take many years to get going in the ground, which is why this vegetable is so much more expensive than others. A good source of all the B-complex vitamins, vitamins C, E and K, asparagus also contains useful amounts of iron, zinc and selenium. Rich in the antioxidant glutathione, asparagus has a long-standing reputation as an efficient liver cleanser. A natural diuretic, it also contains inulin, a prebiotic that supports the beneficial bacteria in the gut. The only downside to asparagus (apart from it being quite pricey) is the way its sulphurous amino acids create smelly wee!

Chicory

The ancient Egyptians and the Romans used chicory root and leaves to help liver function and cleanse the blood. Chicory comes from the same leafy lettuce-like family as radicchio, and both are good to eat (see page 32). They are good sources of vitamins C, E and K. Their bitter taste comes from lactucopicrin, an ingredient that has been used in medicine as an anti-malarial as well as a painkiller.

Herbalists may also use dried chicory root and leaves as a tonic for the liver. Some coffee mixes also include ground chicory root for its bitter coffee-like flavour.

Dandelion

We all know this plant with its bright yellow flowers, and it grows almost anywhere. It's considered a weed but in fact it is extremely nutritious and useful, belonging to the same botanical *Asteraceae* family as artichokes and milk thistle. The leaves are rich in vitamins C, E and – notably – K, as well as beta-carotene, iron and calcium, and are renowned as good for the digestion and the liver and kidneys. The root can also be used, and roasted dandelion root is an easy-to-make, bitter coffee substitute. Dandelion is available as a dried herb for making tisanes, as a tincture and in tablet form, and of course you can gather fresh leaves yourself. Choose tender, young leaves and take care to pick them away from busy roads and other pollution (including dog wee …).

Milk thistle

One of my favourites is milk thistle, also known as silymarin, which grows in southern and western Europe and in North America. The plant has long been used by herbalists to detoxify the liver and treat liver problems. The leaves have white markings and also exude a milky sap when broken – the reason for the plant's common name. The seeds are rich in flavonoids and are the part most commonly used for medicine, but the leaves and flowers can also be eaten. Milk thistle is available as a dried herb, a herbal tincture and in tablet or capsule form. It's also an excellent herbal helper if you should happen to have a hangover …

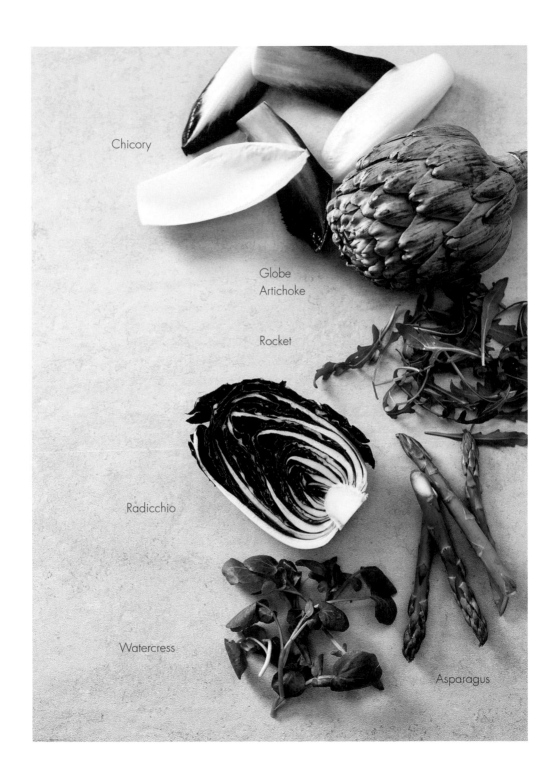

Chicory

Globe
Artichoke

Rocket

Radicchio

Watercress

Asparagus

⑤ Outside: Have a sitz bath

I know this is going to sound weird, but a sitz bath is great for your general health and your skin. The idea is that the cold water 'shocks' the liver into activity, cleansing the body from within. It may seem a bit eccentric, but it really does work. Be warned though – DON'T have a sitz bath if you have a weak heart. The name 'sitz' comes from the German sitzen, meaning sit, and sitting is just what you do – only in cold water.

To take a sitz bath, run a bath with cold water to a depth of about 5cm. Undress, but wear a cardigan or shawl on your top half to keep you warm. Carefully position yourself in the bath with your bottom half in the water and your legs over the side. The water should come up to your navel, covering the liver area. Stay there for 3–5 minutes, then get out of the bath and pat your skin dry. Now snuggle down under your duvet and have a rest.

Liver wrap
Another simple way of detoxifying the liver is to try a 'liver wrap'. All you need is a nice warm hot water bottle, a cold damp flannel and a towel. Make sure you have everything to hand, undress and put on a cosy dressing gown, then lie down somewhere quiet and comfortable.

Put the cold damp flannel on the right-hand side of your body just below the rib cage so it covers your liver area. Your body will respond to the coldness by increasing the circulation in that area. Then place the hot-water bottle on top of the flannel. This will boost blood flow to the liver and help the detoxification process. Put the towel over the hot water bottle and relax for 30 minutes or longer – drop off to sleep if you like – and let nature get to work.

⑥ Inside: Eat and drink foods to cleanse your liver

As well as using plants and herbs to detoxify and support your liver (see pages 29–30), you can include liver-cleansing juices and foods in your diet. Here are a few ideas.

Carrot juice does an excellent job of restoring and cleansing the liver. Part of the liver's job is to deal with fats and oils, and carrot juice helps to reduce the damaging fats and cholesterol levels in the blood. It also keeps our eyes bright and our skin clear. Besides containing many antioxidants, carrots also contain many of the B vitamins, calcium, iron, potassium, sodium and phosphorus – just don't overdo it, as the high levels of beta-carotene in carrots can temporarily give skin an orangey tint.

Kale, beetroot and parsley juice is another good, highly nutritious, liver-friendly juice. Add a little celery and lemon for flavour.

Bitter leaves such as dandelions, watercress, chicory, radicchio and rocket have a high beta-carotene content and are also a rich source of vitamin C, potassium, magnesium, calcium, sodium and iron. Use them to make a powerful liver-cleansing salad, and add some asparagus and artichoke hearts – also good for the liver.

Nettles are not only full of vitamins and good for the liver, but they're also free for you to gather whenever you like. Avoid those by busy roadsides or in fields sprayed with pesticides, and wear gloves when you pick them to avoid their sting. (They don't sting once cooked.) Use nettles like spinach to make a fantastic soup or a pesto-like pasta sauce.

Globe artichokes make an easy and delicious starter. Simply boil the artichokes and serve with some good olive oil or vinaigrette dressing for dunking the leaves before nibbling their tasty tips. Keep the cooking water and use as a base for nutritious soups and smoothies.

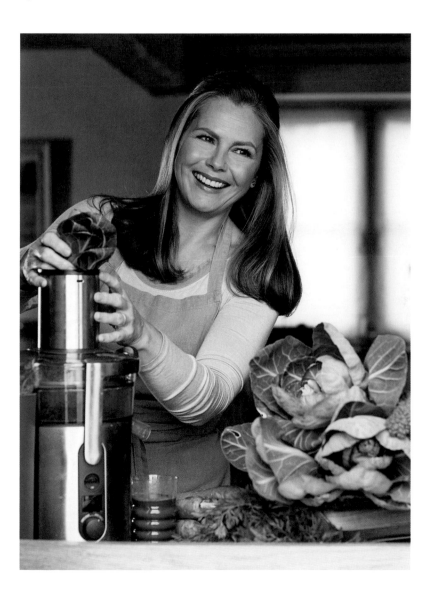

⑦ Outside: Have a herbal steam

A herbal steam is a great weekly treat for your skin. The moisture helps plump up dry or mature skin, and if you have oily skin the heat gently softens blackheads so they are easier to remove. It's simple to do and all you need is a bowl, a towel and some herbs or essential oil. Note: steams are not suitable for those with rosacea, broken veins or very high colour on their cheeks.

- Thoroughly cleanse and exfoliate your skin with a pure cotton cloth or flannel and tie your hair back off your face.

- Fill a bowl with just-boiled water and leave it to cool for a moment or two – you don't want the water to be so hot that it scalds your skin.

- Add a few drops of essential oil or a sprinkling of herbs to the water (see right) and stir them in quickly with a wooden spoon or a toothbrush handle.

- Lean over the bowl, and put a large towel over your head and neck to form a tent to keep in the steam. Close your eyes and take deep breaths through your mouth.

- Move your head around slightly to make sure your whole face is exposed to the steam.

- After 2–3 minutes, take the towel off and pat your face dry.

- Remove any blackheads or small spots using index fingers wrapped in a clean tissue when your face is dry. A magnifying mirror is helpful here.

- Sprinkle cooling toner on to a cotton wool pad and wipe it over your face to soothe the skin. Alternatively, spritz with rose or orange-flower water.

- Follow with your favourite moisturiser.

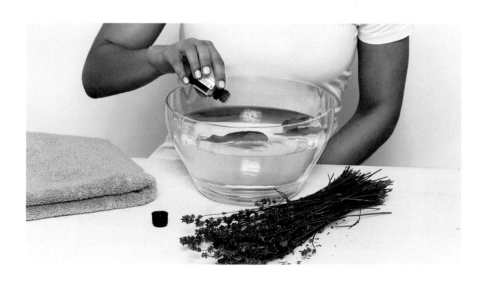

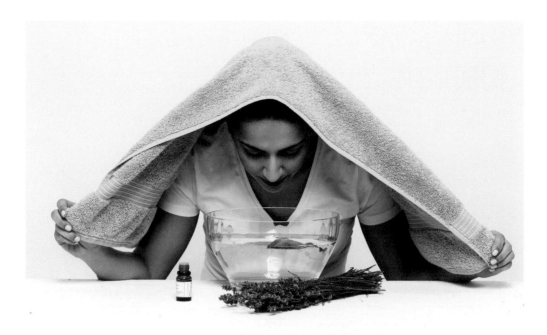

Herbal steams

For normal skin: Lavender and Sage

Ideally, use a few drops of pure lavender essential oil and add 2–3 fresh sage leaves, lightly crushed to release their aromatic oils. Both lavender and sage are a gentle antiseptic and calming, and will help revive tired-looking skin. Dried lavender and sage can also be used, but cover the bowl and leave them to steep for a few minutes to allow them to fully infuse.

For oily and combination skin: Mint and Lemon Peel

Mint makes a great tonic for skin that tends to be on the oily side, while fresh lemon peel is packed with zingy, purifying essential oils. Simply infuse a small handful of fresh (or dried) mint leaves with some strips of fresh, unwaxed lemon peel (use a peeler or lemon zester).

For mature, dry and sensitive skin: Camomile and Rose

Camomile flowers have soothing and skin-calming properties. (If you can't find the dried flowers, simply use a camomile teabag instead.) Infuse for 1 minute before steaming, allowing most of the heat to dissipate, as dry, fragile skins benefit from gentler steaming. Adding a few drops of pure rose oil makes this a really gorgeous, indulgent skin treat. Otherwise, you can use rose water or even freshly picked rose petals.

WEEK THREE:
Healing

This week is about healing and balance – soothing inflamed skin and helping to ease troubled skin or conditions such as eczema and rosacea. And it's a good opportunity to think about how what we're taking into our body (both in terms of food and nutritional supplements) can improve our skin. Skin-calming foods include soothing avocado, packed with vitamin E and beneficial fats, as well as herbal healers such as garlic and ginger.

Try my Baked Avocado Eggs (page 109) as well as the fabulous Garlic and Ginger Mushrooms with Sprouting Broccoli (page 174). Avoid sugary foods as these can increase skin inflammation – if you fancy a sweet treat, try my Quick Banana Ice Cream (page 223) made with no added sugar, yet satisfies the sugar craving.

1 Inside: Eat calming foods to restore your balance

Balance is vital when it comes to what we eat – making sure we have a wide range of foods in sensible proportions. A useful part of this can be maintaining the right acid/alkaline balance in the body. This was an idea originally devised by doctors to help prevent kidney stones and urine infections by using diet to adjust the acidity levels in urine, and many naturopaths also think that eating too many acid-producing foods can lead to weight gain and make a number of conditions such as arthritis, tiredness and osteoporosis worse. What's more, a diet high in acid-producing foods is not good for our skin, as it can cause irritation and inflammation.

That's not to say that all acid-forming foods are unhealthy: they're not. Meat, poultry, fish, pulses and cheese are all reputedly acid-forming, but they're also good sources of protein and we need them in our diet. We just need to make sure we eat enough of the alkalising foods to get the right balance.

The simplest way of achieving this, and doing our skin and our general health a favour, is to eat plenty of fresh vegetables and some fruit. Have a reasonable amount of protein, such as meat, fish and dairy, but restrict refined sugars, alcohol and highly processed foods – all of which are thought to be acid-forming. Some experts suggest a ratio of 70 per cent alkaline foods to 30 per cent acid-forming foods, while others prefer 80/20, but if you eat plenty of fruit and vegetables (especially green veggies), you'll most likely keep your body in a healthy state of balance.

ACID AND ALKALINE FOODS

HIGHLY ALKALINE	MEDIUM ALKALINE	MILDLY ALKALINE	MILDLY ACIDIC	MEDIUM ACIDIC	HIGHLY ACIDIC
Barley grass	Alfalfa	Almonds	Apple cider	Brown rice	Beef
Cucumber	Avocado	Almond butter	vinegar	Cheese	Beer
Dandelion	Beetroot (fresh)	Artichokes	Apples	Chicken	Black tea
Kale	Butter beans	Asparagus	Apricots (fresh	Cereals	Cakes and
Soy lecithin	(dried)	Aubergine	and dried)	(shop-bought)	biscuits
Sprouted seeds	Celery	Banana (ripe)	Blackberries	Eggs	(shop-bought)
Wheat grass	Coriander	Basil	Blueberries	Fish	Coffee
	Endive	Brussels sprouts	Brazil nuts	Milk	Crisps
	Garlic	Buckwheat	Bulgur wheat	(pasteurised)	Croissants
	Ginger	Carrot	Butter	Peanuts and	Fried foods
	Haricot beans	Cauliflower	Cantaloupe	peanut butter	Ice cream
	(dried)	Coconut (fresh)	melon	Pineapple	Lamb
	Natural fruit	Coconut oil	Cashews	Pistachios	Pickled
	juice	Courgettes	Clementines	Pomegranate	vegetables
	Radishes	Cumin seeds	Couscous	Raspberry	Pork
	Sorrel	Fennel seeds	Dates (fresh and	Sourdough	Spirits
	Spinach	Figs (dried and	dried)	bread	Sugar
		fresh)	Flax seeds	Wheat	Sweetened fruit
		Flaxseed oil	Green tea	Wine	juice
		Grapefruit	Hazelnuts	Yoghurt	Sweeteners
		Green cabbage	Honey	(sweetened)	(artificial)
		Green tea	Mango		White flour
		Herbal tea	Maple syrup		
		Lambs lettuce	Milk (un-		
		Leeks	pasteurised)		
		Lemon (fresh)	Nectarine		
		Lentils	Oats		
		Lettuce	Orange		
		Lime	Peach		
		Olive oil	Pear		
		Onion	Pumpkin seeds		
		Parsnip	Rye bread		
		Peas	Strawberries		
		Peppers	Sunflower seeds		
		Pine nuts	Sweet potatoes		
		Potatoes	Walnuts		
		Red cabbage	Wholemeal		
		Savoy cabbage	bread		
		Seaweed	Yoghurt		
		Sesame oil	(unsweetened)		
		Sesame seeds			
		Spelt			
		Spinach			
		Tomatoes			
		Turnip			
		Watercress			

Drinking juices and smoothies – preferably ones you make yourself – is a great way of increasing your intake of beneficial nutrients. And it's best to use more vegetables than fruit in your juices, too, as they're lower in natural sugars. By the way, you may be surprised to learn that foods you might think of as 'acid', such as lemons, limes and grapefruit, actually have an alkalising effect on the body – as long as they are freshly squeezed from the fruit and not heat-treated or pasteurised.

Alkaline Skin Smoothie

Serves 1

1 small beetroot

1 banana, peeled

1 tbsp ground almonds

150ml almond or rice milk

Juice the beetroot, then add all ingredients to a blender or food processor and whizz until smooth. You can also use bottled beetroot.

Alkaline Greenie Glow Juice

Serves 1

1 pink grapefruit, peeled

3 handfuls washed spinach

3 small asparagus spears

2 celery sticks

Simply juice and serve!

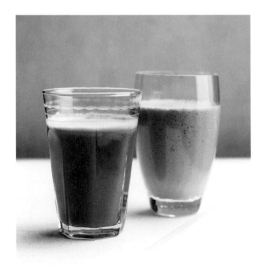

② Outside: How to calm skin inflammations such as eczema and rosacea

Eczema

Eczema is a non-contagious skin condition that's characterised by patches of hot, itchy, scaly skin which can appear anywhere on the body. The skin may produce weeping blisters and discharge, and if scratched may become raw and bleed. It's important to mention that if you're suffering from severe eczema you must get medical treatment, so do check with your doctor. There is, though, a great deal you can do to help reduce its severity.

- Take extra care to check the ingredients in products you use on your skin. Use unfragranced toiletries (even natural essential oils can aggravate) and definitely avoid anything that contains sodium lauryl/laureth sulphate (SLS), which makes eczema worse.

- When bathing or showering, don't have the water too hot. Use an emollient wash (unfragranced, from the chemist) instead of soap or foaming gels.

- If you use perfume, spray it on your hair or your clothes, not on your skin.

- Be aware of what you eat and note any reactions. Consider getting screening for food allergies that are common triggers for eczema. Those with eczema may find they can't drink ordinary cow's milk, but are fine with organic cow's milk. This may be because of the higher Omega-3 content of the milk, possibly due to the natural red clover in the cow's forage.

- Make sure you have plenty of plant oils and essential fatty acids (EFAs) in your diet. EFAs help to restore lipid levels in the outer cells of the skin, and so prevent flaking and dryness.

- They are also natural anti-inflammatories. Excellent sources are evening primrose oil (such as Rigel seed), borage seed (starflower) oil, flaxseed oil and hemp seed oil.

- Use soothing creams containing the oils mentioned above, which can ease inflammation of the skin. Products containing manuka honey can also help – high-strength manuka honey has antibacterial and anti-inflammatory properties and is useful for soothing the skin.

- Choose creams that are properly preserved. Eczema and other skin conditions can be made worse by creams that have become contaminated by bacteria. Phenoxyethanol can irritate those with eczema.

- House dust contains dust mite droppings, which can trigger eczema attacks, so vacuum carefully and regularly. Wash bedding weekly on a hot wash cycle and air daily.

- Use gentle household cleaners and avoid those with harsh chemicals and strong scents, as these can also be irritants.

Rosacea

This is another common, non-contagious skin condition, which causes the face to flush and turn red, sometimes with small red spots and a burning, itching sensation.

No one yet understands quite what causes rosacea, but triggers include exposure to extreme weather, hot sun, alcohol, spicy food, stress and heavy exercise. There's no permanent cure, but treatment can help to control the condition and your GP can prescribe antibiotics or gels and creams that will help to ease symptoms. There are also a few ways you can help yourself.

- Try to identify triggers and avoid them where possible.

- Be sure to include plant oils and essential fatty acids in your diet. Probiotics, such as *Acidophilus* in live yoghurt, can help boost the 'good' bacteria in the gut, helping the body get rid of compounds that may cause inflammation.

- Don't use exfoliating creams, as they can make your skin even more sensitive.

- Avoid saunas and steam rooms – the high temperatures will aggravate your skin. If your face feels hot after vigorous exercise, splash it with cool water or use a cool flannel.

- Sun is a common trigger for rosacea sufferers, so use a good mineral-based (not synthetic chemical) sunscreen, made with minerals such as zinc or titanium dioxide. It should have an SPF of 15 or higher and protect against both UVA and UVB rays. Ideally, stay in the shade and cover up with clothing and a wide-brimmed hat.

- Use skincare products that contain naturally skin-calming ingredients. Botanicals such as aloe vera, calendula and cucumber are good, but fragrance (including natural essential oils), alcohol, clove oil, menthol, tea tree oil and witch hazel can aggravate.

- Creams or ointments containing one or more of the following have been shown to help rosacea: Chrysanthellum indicum, green tea, liquorice and niacinamide (a form of Vitamin B3).

Skin-calming foods can help. The recipe below is one of my all-time favourite skin drinks – a velvety smoothie-style skin-calming juice.

For Eczema/Psoriasis/Rosacea

1 large carrot
½ fennel bulb
¼ medium cucumber

½ ripe avocado, stoned
1 borage seed oil or evening primrose oil capsule (such as Rigel seed)

Juice the carrot, fennel and cucumber in a juicer before placing the combined juices in a blender. Add the avocado and the contents of the oil capsule. Whizz until smooth.

③ Inside: Eat healing skin-friendly foods

Our skin, just like the rest of our body, responds to what we eat. So eating well is of prime importance if we're to maintain a radiant glow from top to toe. Make sure you have a good balance of protein, vegetables, fruit, and fats – but keep away from refined sugars. Not only does sugar pile on the pounds, it's also a real enemy of the skin. It increases inflammation and contributes to skin ageing, so avoid it as much as you can. Your skin will thank you.

Protein

Essential for healthy skin, hair and nails, as well as the rest of the body. The amino acids in proteins are the 'building blocks' of the body, and although technically we can obtain the nutrients we need from plant sources, complete proteins come mainly from animal sources, such as meat, game, fish, dairy and eggs. Try to include small amounts of protein in every main meal. Don't forget that nuts and seeds are also a good source of protein, so include these in your diet, too.

Vegetables and fruit

These contain loads of vitamins and minerals as well as the fibre that's vital for keeping our elimination system working and expelling the daily digestive waste matter that can damage health and skin. Aim to eat at least five portions a day – but more is even better. Make sure you choose veg in a range of colours – dark green spinach and chard, red peppers and beetroot, and vivid orange carrots, squash and sweet potatoes.

Good fats

Don't be scared to eat good fats. The body – and the brain – needs fat to function properly, and we also need fats to absorb the all-important, skin-friendly fat-soluble vitamins such as A, D, E and K. Good fats include oils such as olive, rapeseed, avocado and nut oils, oily fish, and nuts and seeds (which also contain lots of skin-building nutrients).

Milk is important too, but go for whole milk. It's a myth that semi-skimmed or skimmed milk is better for us – whole milk is only 3.5 per cent fat, so is not a high-fat food and is a rich source of goodness. Try to buy organic milk where possible, and look for the words 'pasture-fed' on the label. Milk from cows that have grazed on grass as nature intended, instead of being housed 24/7 in barns, may be more nutritious, higher in Omega-3 skin-friendly fats – and better for the environment.

Avoid fats in processed foods, particular hydrogenated fats and trans fats, such as hardened vegetable (palm) oil. They do us no good at all. And butter is better for us than margarine … just don't eat too much of it!

Grains

Go for non-refined grains – whole brown rice, wholegrain or rye or spelt bread, and wholemeal pasta as well as quinoa, freekeh and spelt. Cut out processed white grains such as those in white bread, shop-bought cakes and biscuits, and other 'fancy goods' made with white sugar and flour. You won't suffer – you'll find plenty of skin-friendly treats to make with the recipes in this book – and your face will look more fabulous for it.

My Top Skin-friendly Foods:

- Almonds
- Avocados
- Beef (grass- or pasture-fed)
- Brown rice (organic, short-grain)
- Dark chocolate, minimum 80 per cent cocoa solids

- Eggs (organic)
- Fish (oily varieties)
- Green leafy vegetables
- Seeds (especially pumpkin and sunflower)
- Yoghurt (plain, live, organic)

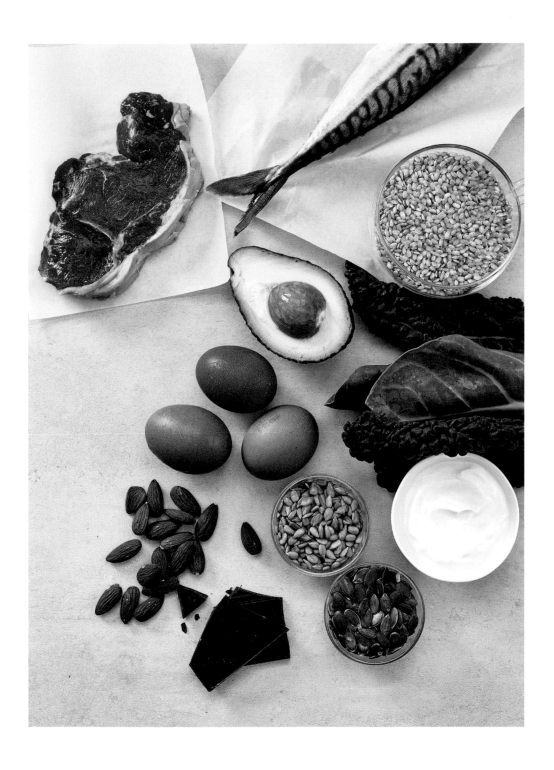

④ Outside: Make a healing face mask

A nourishing facial mask once a week or so is one of the best treats for our skin. It's an excellent way of helping to cleanse skin of impurities, leaving the face beautifully clean and super-soft. Look for a good soothing mask to buy, or you can make your own at home, using the recipe below.

To use the mask, clean your face as usual (see page 24–25). Then smooth the mask over your face and neck, avoiding your eyes, lips and hairline. If you've got any of the mixture left over, give the backs of your hands a treat, too. Leave for 10–15 minutes, then rinse the mask off (use a pure cotton cloth or flannel) and splash your face with cool water.

For a special treat, apply the mask while you're relaxing in a warm bath. The steam from the water vapour will soften your skin and allow the mask to work its magic all the more effectively.

Soothing Face Mask

This simple recipe is one of my classic favourites: a gentle, fruity, home-made face mask that's easy to make, and is excellent for soothing tired, dehydrated skin. Use on the backs of your hands, too.

1 small ripe banana (preferably organic)   5ml runny honey (Manuka is a good option)
25g finely ground oatmeal

Simply mash the banana thoroughly in a small bowl until it forms a smooth paste. Stir in the oatmeal and honey. Mix together well before applying to freshly cleansed skin on the face and neck. Relax for 15–20 minutes before rinsing it off with warm water.

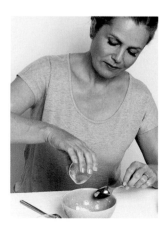
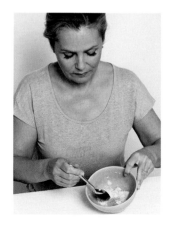
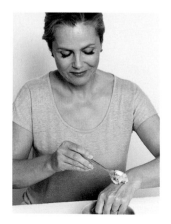

⑤ Inside: Try an anti-acne diet

Acne, with its spots, blackheads and whiteheads, affects too many of us and is very distressing. The wrong foods don't cause acne – the main triggers are hormones and stress – but some foods may make it worse. If your acne is severe you may need antibiotics and it's *really* important to see a doctor, who can prescribe medication for you to prevent permanent skin scarring. Don't be scared of conventional medication – it can be a genuine help. But once treatment is under way, it's well worth having a good look at what you eat and identify what changes you could make. Once conventional medication has stabilised the condition, a good diet with lots of fresh vegetables and healthy probiotics (such as live yoghurt) can help you maintain good skin naturally.

HERE ARE SOME IDEAS:

- Blood sugar swings can cause inflammation, so eat three small meals and two snacks a day to keep levels stable.

- Avoid sugary foods – but you can still enjoy a small amount of antioxidant-rich, very dark chocolate – 70 per cent cocoa solids is best.

- Drink fresh herb or green tea, or chicory instead of coffee. And drink plenty of pure, still water – at least 2 litres a day.

- Try cutting out cow's milk and soya milk, which can aggravate acne for some. Drink no-sugar almond, oat or rice milk instead.

- Try taking vitamins A and D as well as zinc. These can help by stimulating the growth of healthy new skin cells. A daily dose of sunshine (a source of vitamin D) can also help – 20 minutes should suffice. Note that vitamin A supplements are not recommended for pregnant women.

- Treat existing acne lesions with creams such as ActivClear, which contains tea tree essential oil, vitamin A and extracts of the herb tribulus.

- Aim for 7–8 hours of sleep a night, and try to avoid stress. Develop ways of dealing with stressful situations – meditation, yoga and prayer can all help.

- Eating a low-GL (glycemic load) diet also helps stabilise blood sugar – I find it makes me feel so much better, and increases my energy. The glycemic load measures the amount of carbohydrate in a serving of food and how quickly it raises blood sugar levels. Experts believe this provides a better guide as to the effect a food will have on blood sugar. Foods with a low GL (below 10) provide less of a spike in blood sugar levels. Foods with a GL of 10–20 are considered medium GL, and those over 20 are high GL. The chart on page 46 shows the glycemic loads of a selection of foods.

GLYCEMIC LOAD TABLE

FOOD	PORTION	GL
VEGETABLES		

Most vegetables are low in carbohydrate so are low GL

FOOD	PORTION	GL
Beetroot	80g	5
Broad beans	80g	9
Carrot	80g	1
Parsnip	80g	12
Peas	80g	4
Sweetcorn	80g	11

FRUIT

FOOD	PORTION	GL
Apple	120g	6
Apricots (dried)	60g	8
Banana	120g	15
Blueberries	80g	3
Cherries	120g	3
Dates (dried)	30g	12
Figs (dried)	20g	6
Grapes	120g	10
Grapefruit	120g	3
Kiwi fruit	120g	6
Mango	120g	8
Orange	120g	5
Peach	120g	5
Pear	120g	4
Pineapple	120g	5
Plums	120g	5
Prunes	30g	3
Strawberries	120g	1
Watermelon	120g	4

FISH AND MEAT

No carbs so no GI/GL

DAIRY

FOOD	PORTION	GL
Milk, whole	250g	3
Yoghurt, plain	200g	3
Ice cream	50g	6

OILS AND FATS

No carbs so no GI/GL

NUTS AND SEEDS

Almonds, brazil nuts, hazelnuts, walnuts, pumpkin seeds, sesame seeds are all low in carbs so no GI/GL

FOOD	PORTION	GL
Cashew nuts	50g	3
Peanuts	50g	1
Popcorn	20g	8

PULSES

FOOD	PORTION	GL
Black-eyed beans	150g	13
Butter beans (cooked)	150g	6
Chickpeas (cooked)	150g	8
Haricot beans (cooked)	150g	12
Lentils (cooked)	150g	5
Red kidney beans	150g	8

STARCHY CARBOHYDRATES

FOOD	PORTION	GL
Bread (wholemeal)	30g	9
Bulgur wheat (cooked)	150g	12
Couscous (cooked)	150g	23
Muesli	30g	10
Porridge (cooked)	250g	13
Potato (baked)	150g	18
Potatoes, new	150g	12
Quinoa (cooked)	125g	13
Rice, brown (cooked)	150g	18
Rice, white long-grain (cooked)	120g	23
Rye crispbread	25g	11
Spaghetti, white (cooked)	180g	22
Spaghetti, wholemeal (cooked)	180g	17
Sweet potato	150g	22

EXTRAS

FOOD	PORTION	GL
Dark chocolate	15g	4
Honey	25g	12
Maple syrup	1 tbsp	7

⑥ Outside: Run yourself a healing herbal bath

I find that a lovely long soak in a warm bath is one of the nicest ways to relax and recover after a stressful day. And if you add a few extras to the water, a bath can also help heal and soothe your skin. Try some of these naturally skin-soothing ideas for a bit of bath-time bliss.

Herbal Bath

A simple way of adding herbs to your bath is to put them in a muslin square, tie it tightly at the top and hang it from the tap so it dangles in the running water. This way you don't have to pick out lots of bits of herb out of the bath when you're done. If you don't have any muslin, try cutting off the foot section of a pair of tights or stockings instead. Or, you can simply throw in some herbal tea bags! The best herbs for calming and soothing the skin are camomile, lavender, yarrow and marigold.

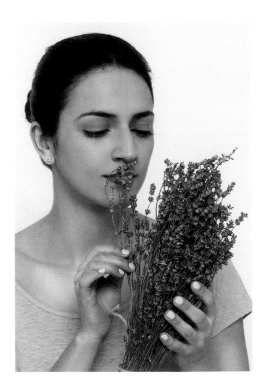

Milk Bath

Add 1 tablespoon of dried milk powder to your warm bath, and you will emerge with beautifully soft skin.

Olive Oil Bath

Add 2 teaspoons of olive, rapeseed or sunflower oil or 1 teaspoonful of coconut oil to the water for another way to soften your skin. Take care, though, as the oil can make the sides of the bath very slippery.

Salt and Seaweed Bath

To help soothe itchy or inflamed skin, add a little Dead Sea salt (particularly rich in minerals such as iodine) or ordinary sea salt and a pinch of culinary seaweed to your bath.

Epsom Salts Bath

Epsom salts are cheap to buy and have a soothing effect on the skin. Studies have shown that the body absorbs small amounts of magnesium from the salts, which may also help ease aches and pains. Use at least 2 cupfuls for the best effect, and soak for 10–15 minutes.

Oatmeal Bath

Whizz up some porridge oats in your blender until you have a fine powder, and pile this into a muslin bag (see above). Put the bag into the bath while the water is running to help soothe and calm irritated skin. Add a few drops of lavender essential oil for a gorgeous scent.

⑦ Inside: Consider taking skin supplements

Our skin needs nutrients to repair itself and reproduce. A good, well-balanced diet should provide the supplies our skin needs, but farming techniques and food processing can destroy many of the nutrients in food before it even reaches our plate. And in our busy lives, it can be hard to make sure that we get all our much-needed minerals and vitamins, so taking supplements can help us top up. Here are some suggestions that can help skin glow. **Note:** Always follow the maker's instructions for the dosage and when to take supplements. If you're pregnant, have a medical condition or you're taking prescription drugs, always check with your doctor before taking supplements.

Essential fatty acids

EFAs are vital components of all cell membranes and play a vital role in keeping skin healthy. Consider taking an EFA supplement with Omega-3 and GLA (gamma-linoleic acid). GLA is an Omega-6 fatty acid found in plant-based oils such as borage seed and evening primrose oil (such as Rigel seed).

Vitamins and minerals

A good multi-vitamin formula tops you up with skin-saving nutrients and can help 'plug the gap' with any shortfall.

Vitamin E

If you're concerned about ageing skin, consider taking a supplement containing at least 50mg of vitamin E. Make sure it is from a natural source, not synthetically produced, as this is less effective. Natural vitamin E will be listed as 'd-alpha-tocopherol' while the synthetic type is called 'dl-alpha-tocopherol'. You can remember this by: dl = delivers less.

Chlorella

Chlorella is a green algae packed with protein, vitamins and minerals and is great for nourishing the skin. It is also reputed to de-acidify the gut, so may help alkalise the body. Chlorella is also a fabulous source of chlorophyll, which helps cleanse the system. Chlorella can be taken as a powder – add some to a smoothie – or in tablet form, and with regular use you should find your skin starts to appear plumper and healthier. Chlorophyll, by the way, is what gives plants their green colour and enables them to photosynthesise.

Collagen

Collagen is a protein and makes up about 65 per cent of our skin, giving it resilience, tone and stretch, but as we grow older production in the body decreases, so contributing to the ageing of our skin. Look into taking collagen supplements to help maintain youthful-looking skin. These are made from hydrolised collagen protein (a more absorbable form) and come from either beef gelatine or fish skin proteins.

Probiotics

Probiotics are an excellent way for us to maintain good digestive health as well as helping to keep the skin clear. They're present in live yoghurt, fermented foods and drinks such as kefir, but you can also take them as supplements. Some of the best to look for are *Lactobacillus acidophilus, L. paracasei, L. plantarum, L. casei, L. lactis and L. rhamnosus; Bifidobacterium bifidum, B. breve, B. longum and B. lactis.*

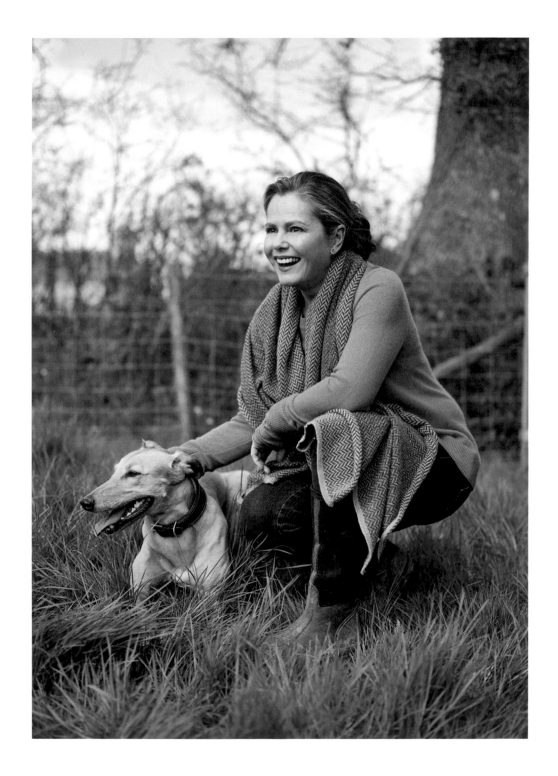

WEEK FOUR:
Nourishing

This week is all about how best to feed our skin to achieve a more youthful radiance. What we put on our skin is important, but no skin cream can make up for a poor diet. Our skin, just like the rest of our body, needs plenty of vitamins, minerals and essential fatty acids in the form of good food. Some of our best internal moisturisers come from nutrient-dense foods, including nuts, seeds and oily fish.

Don't miss my Bircher Breakfast to nourish the skin from within (page 97) as well as plenty of oily fish enriched dishes, including Smoked Mackerel with Poppy Seed Salad (page 151) and Salmon Fishcakes (page 193) made without potato to be far more skin-friendly.

➊ Outside: Moisturise your skin

The route to healthy, youthful-looking skin is simple. First, we need to feed our skin from the inside with a nourishing diet. And second, keep to a proper skincare routine, one of the most important parts of which is moisturising.

The skin makes its own moisture in the form of sebum, but it struggles to combat the effects of wind, sun, central heating and air-conditioning, all of which are dehydrating. Smoking, alcohol and a poor diet also have a negative effect. In addition, the skin's ability to retain moisture reduces with age, so our need for moisturiser increases.

All sorts of extravagant claims are made by some moisturisers – we're told they will stop our skin ageing or banish wrinkles. But they could only do this by changing the physical structure of the skin. Any cream that could dramatically do that would have to be classed as a drug, and would only be available from a doctor on prescription (such as Retin-A, used to treat acne and skin discolouration).

What a moisturiser can do is nourish and protect the upper layers of the skin and slow down the ageing process. It tops up the skin's moisture content by forming a film over the surface, and so combats water loss. Dermatologists (skin doctors) refer to this as trans-epidermal water loss, or TWL, and it is used as a measure of how much moisture is passed through the body and out of the skin. One of the most important functions of a moisturiser is to reduce or slow TWL, so our skin stays well hydrated and smooth-looking, as well as feeling more comfortable. All skin types benefit from a good moisturiser as these creams can also help to regulate oil production.

When choosing a moisturiser, be guided by how the product feels on your skin. A good product should be easily absorbed and not leave your skin feeling greasy. Look for one containing plenty of genuinely skin-friendly ingredients such as essential fatty acids (EFAs), vitamins and botanical extracts. Plant oils provide a more skin-compatible base than mineral oils (avoid liquid paraffin or mineral oil on the label). Natural plant-based ingredients such as avocado oil and shea butter have added benefits, such as vitamins, and are well known for their protective and nourishing properties.

Read the label on the product carefully (see page 14 for more on understanding labels). It's up to you whether you go for a cream, lotion or oil – whatever feels best. But in general slightly thicker, richer moisturisers are good for drier skins, while those with oily skin are better off with a more fluid product that gives a more matt effect on the skin. If you have very sensitive skin, avoid fragranced moisturisers, even natural essential oils.

Always apply moisturiser to scrupulously clean skin. And don't forget to take it down to your neck and cleavage – it is no good having a youthful-looking face and a wrinkly neck! It's also a good idea to massage any excess into the backs of your hands.

EYE CREAM

The delicate skin around our eyes is often the first to show lines, and eye creams aim to diminish these wrinkles and reduce puffiness. They usually contain similar ingredients to facial moisturisers, but these may be more concentrated and will have been ophthalmically tested to ensure that they don't irritate the sensitive eye area. A good eye cream should be quite light and quickly absorbed so it doesn't leave a greasy film.

NIGHT CREAM/DAY CREAM

I'm happy to use the same moisturiser night and morning, although many ranges have different formulas, with a richer cream to use at night. However, some beauty therapists will say that using a richer cream around the eyes at night can cause puffiness in the morning. My preference is to apply a serum or facial oil at night to give my skin an overnight boost. The price tags can vary wildly, so to get the best value for money it really is worth learning how to read the labels.

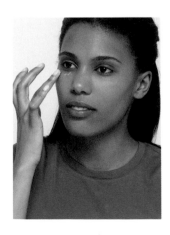
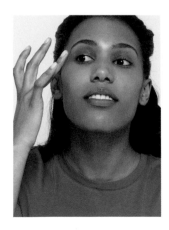
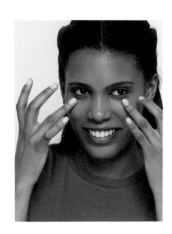

Ingredients to look for in a moisturiser

Most of my favourite skincare ingredients come from the natural world and many from the plant kingdom. Not only are they often more compatible with the skin than their lab-made synthetic counterparts, they often contain useful skin-boosting ingredients such as antioxidants and anti-inflammatory compounds.

Rosehip oil is extracted from the beautiful orangey-red rosehips you see in the hedgerows. A thick, greenish-gold colour, this oil is rich in antioxidants and EFAs and is one of my favourite moisturising ingredients. Clinical studies show that it can soften scar tissue, reduce 'age' spots and improve the appearance of fine surface facial lines. It's an excellent facial massage oil, on its own or in blends.

Avocado oil is a good source of vitamins A (in the form of beta-carotene), B-complex, D and E, and I believe it's one of the best plant oils for soothing dry skin. It is also a good source of linoleic acid, which helps strengthen the membranes surrounding skin.

Vitamin E is a particularly important ingredient in creams for the mature skin because of its ability to help combat the free-radical cell damage that contributes to skin ageing. Look for moisturisers containing the natural, rather than the synthetic, form of vitamin E, as it is about a third more potent.

Argan oil is another personal favourite of mine and comes from a tree that grows along the coastal regions of Morocco. Rich in vitamin E, it is highly prized by the Berber people, who use it to help protect their skin from the dry desert winds and strong sun. Scientists are still looking into the unique plant sterols contained in argan oil, and research shows it to be both anti-inflammatory and restorative.

Borage oil contains high levels of gamma-linoleic acid (GLA), an essential fatty acid that's linked to skin-cell strengthening and increased TWL and retained moisture levels.

Shea butter is a fantastic natural moisturiser for all skin types. Extracted from the nuts housed inside the chestnut-like fruit of the shea tree, shea butter contains an abundance of useful EFAs, as well as beta-carotene and natural-source vitamin E.

Cacay oil is a relatively recent discovery, and it seems to have some excellent properties. It comes from the nut of a tree that grows wild along the base of the Andes Mountains in South America, and has long been used by local people there. A beautiful golden oil, it's particularly rich in the natural form of vitamin E and retinol – an ingredient that may help to reduce wrinkles and scarring, delay the signs of ageing and generally plump up the skin. It is expensive but you only need to use a few drops, massaged into your skin the last thing each night. Look for sustainable brands that support local communities in their harvesting.

② Inside: Make sure you include plenty of plant oils in your diet

A well-balanced diet will help to ensure that your skin gets all the supplies it needs, and some of the most nutritious and skin-friendly foods are plant oils. You may link the word 'oil' with fattening, high-calorie food, but if you choose a few drops of the right oils they do you nothing but good. Eating good oils can actually help weight loss by boosting the metabolism and helping the body burn energy faster. Many oils are an excellent source of vitamins and essential fatty acids, and they're vital for the healthy functioning of our whole body.

Fats and oils have become a hot topic in recent years, where we've been bombarded with ads for 'fat-free' foods, and terms such as 'polyunsaturates' and 'trans fats' are bandied about on labels. The truth is that we need some fats in our diet, but we need fats from unprocessed, natural foods.

Saturated fats mostly come from animals and include lard, butter and cheese. They're generally solid. There are two forms of plant-based saturated fats and these are coconut oil and palm oil.

Unsaturated fats can be monounsaturated or polyunsaturated, and they are found in plant oils. Polyunsaturates contain essential fatty acids Omega-3 and Omega-6, which we know are so important for skin health as well as general wellbeing. They are called 'essential' because our body needs these fats but cannot make them. We have to get them from food.

To get the benefits of plant oils, it's important to choose the right kinds and always look for the words 'natural', 'unrefined' and 'cold-pressed' on the label. Cold-pressed means exactly what it says – the nuts or seeds are ground, then pressed to release the oil. In more commercial methods the oil is heated before pressing, which helps to release more oil. Chemical solvents may also be used to get more from the nuts and seed pods. Unfortunately, this can also destroy some of the valuable nutrients. Other cooking oils are put through an even more destructive process in which the oils are highly refined, resulting in a devitalised product, lacking in the wonderful benefits of natural oils. Cold-pressed oils cost more because they are more expensive to produce, but they are usually worth it.

WHEN BUYING OILS, HERE ARE A FEW TIPS

- Look for darker oils with a good nutty smell – refined oils are bleached and deodorised.

- Choose oils packaged in metal tins or dark bottles – exposure to the light makes oil turn rancid more quickly.

- To be sure of what you're getting, choose oils from a single source, rather than blends from different countries and/or varieties.

- Check best before dates, and store your oil in a cool dark place.

Enjoying oils

Oils are most nutritious – and skin friendly – when unheated. I like to make sure I have a tablespoon of good-quality, uncooked oil every day. This can be in a salad dressing, drizzled over vegetables or a bowl of soup, or added to a smoothie. Dips such as hummus (see page 122) are another good way of consuming oil, and they make a perfect pick-me-up snack when hunger pangs strike. One of my very favourite ways of enjoying a good olive oil is to pour some into a little bowl, then dunk a hunk of good bread into it. Delicious.

Cooking with oil

In years gone by, we cooked with animal fats such as dripping and lard, but in recent years the advice has been to avoid these and go for vegetable oils instead. But these aren't without their problems, especially the more common, polyunsaturated kind.

When polyunsaturated oils are heated they lose nutrients, but they also undergo other changes and can produce free-radicals and other toxic compounds. These molecular fragments have been linked to cell damage and all sorts of conditions, from cancer to skin ageing.

The different structures of oils mean that some are more stable than others at high temperatures. The least stable are polyunsaturated sunflower, safflower, soybean and corn (maize) oil. More stable options for cooking are the mono-unsaturated oils including rapeseed (canola) and olive oil.

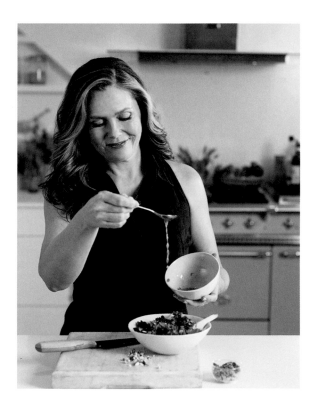

Some of my favourite oils for use in cooking

Olive oil is the best of all oils to my mind. It tastes wonderful and has a multitude of proven nutritional and health benefits. It's at its best unheated for dressings and drizzling, but can be used for cooking – though not at high temperatures, such as in frying. Use the darker 'extra virgin' kind for tasty dressings, and the less expensive, lighter 'pure' version for cooking. Keep in a cool dark place, but not in the fridge as it will solidify when cold.

Rapeseed or canola oil is a light oil with a neutral flavour that is good for cooking. It goes rancid quickly and is best stored in the fridge. This is a favourite of mine.

Pumpkin seed oil has a lovely dark green colour and a good flavour. I adore it in dressings (see pages 236–237) or drizzled over pasta or rice. It's almost a meal in itself!

Walnut oil has a lovely, strong, nutty taste and makes a delicious dressing. You can use it on its own or add a few drops to a lighter oil, such as rapeseed, for extra flavour.

Flaxseed oil is less familiar to many of us, but its healing benefits have been admired for thousands of years. Although a polyunsaturated oil, it's unusually rich in Omega-3 fatty acids and can be helpful for the skin, particularly for inflammatory skin conditions. Its nutrients are easily destroyed by light and heat so it should be stored in the fridge. This is not one to use for cooking, but it's great for drizzling or for adding a spoonful to a smoothie or juice.

Sesame oil has a strong flavour and responds well to heating, so it can be used in dishes such as stir-fries. Avoid 'toasted' sesame oil, which has had its structure damaged by over-heating.

Avocado oil is rich in plant sterols, essential fatty acids and vitamin E. Avocados are generally eaten as the whole fruit, but the oil is also delicious and wonderful in dressings.

Coconut oil differs from all the above as it is a saturated plant fat and comes in solid form. It's rich in essential fatty acids, as well as having a little vitamin E and K. It does have quite a coconutty flavour, so may not work for all recipes (unless you love coconut). It is also a saturated fat, so it's stable for heating and cooking, but is best used in moderation. It adds a natural sweetness to snacks and sweet treats, too.

③ Outside: Give yourself a facial massage with plant oil

I find that giving myself a facial massage with some nourishing plant oil is a lovely way to have some 'me-time'. It doesn't take long and leaves me feeling wonderfully calm and relaxed. We all tend to hold a lot of tension in our facial muscles (especially if you grind your teeth at night) and this is a good way of helping to release it. What's more – your skin will glow!

Plant oils are found in many good moisturisers and other skin treatments, and help give our skin a wonderful boost. They're easily absorbed into the upper levels of the skin and they're full of skin-friendly nutrients. They help to hold water at the skin's surface, so they have an excellent firming and plumping effect, too.

One of my favourite oils for facial massage is rosehip oil, rich in antioxidants, EFAs and other nutrients, including vitamin C. It also contains a form of vitamin A that helps to remove dead skin cells, revealing a fresher, brighter skin. Other good oils for facial massage are peach kernel, almond and hazelnut. You can also add a drop or two of essential oil for fragrance (unless your skin is very sensitive) – see my suggestion below.

Miracle Massage Blend

This is a wonderful mix of skin-reviving plant oils, and it's so easy to make.

50ml rosehip oil

10ml avocado oil

2 natural-source vitamin E capsules

1 evening primrose oil (such as Rigel seed) or starflower oil capsule

2 drops neroli, lavender and/or rose absolute essential oil

Simply pierce the oil capsules and mix to make the oil blend, then add the fragrance. My favourites are neroli, lavender and rose for my own dry skin, but you can adjust according to personal preference. Juniper and petitgrain are associated with oilier skin types, while frankincense is often used for more mature skins.

- Wash your hands well, then cleanse and tone your face. Pour a few drops of oil into your palm, then rub your hands together to warm the oil. Close your eyes, take a deep breath and hold your palms over your face. Take a few more deep breaths.

- Place one hand on your forehead and put the other on the back of your neck. Press lightly and hold for a minute. Keeping your hands in place, gently rotate your neck. Ease any tight spots at the back of your neck with your fingertips.

- Using both hands, massage the base of your skull. Work around to the back of the ears, into the corners of the jaw and along the jaw line. Repeat six times.

- Shake your shoulders and arms to release any tension. Using the thumb and forefinger of each hand, pinch along your jawline. Work backwards and forwards six times. Using your middle fingers, massage your cheeks to relax any tight spots.

- Press your thumbs against the sides of your nose. Start at the top and work down, smoothing outwards. With the sides of your thumbs, sweep out under each eye socket going from nose to temple. Repeat six times.

- Press along your eyebrows with your index fingers, starting from the top of your nose and working outwards. Repeat six times. Gently sweep your index fingers along your eyebrows, then around the eye socket, giving a final press on the inner eye area. Repeat six times.

- Using your fingertips, lightly tap over your whole face. Start at the top of the forehead, and work down over the eye area, cheeks and sides of the face to the jawline and chin. Continue to work up and down to stimulate blood flow and oxygenate the skin. Finally sweep your hands across your face and take a few more deep breaths. *Et voilà!*

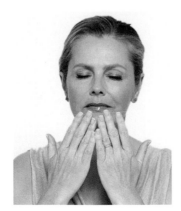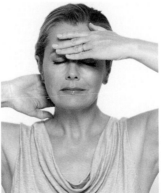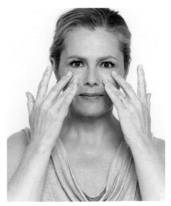

4 Inside: Eat oily fish for skin health

Oily fish, such as herring, mackerel, sardines and – to a lesser extent – salmon and trout, are packed with Omega-3 essential fatty acids (EFAs) and other nutrients, so they're good for our general health and brilliant for our skin. They help to stimulate cell renewal and increase the skin's natural moisture content.

Fish oils may also help inflammatory skin problems such as psoriasis. These EFAs are vital for maintaining healthy skin cells, keeping them healthy and strong. They also encourage the production of strong collagen and elastin fibres in the dermis, helping to prevent wrinkling and sagging.

There are two main groups of essential fatty acids: Omega-3 and Omega-6. It's important to have them in the right balance, which is thought to be a ratio of 2:1 Omega-6 to Omega-3. However, many of us now consume a much higher proportion of Omega-6, largely because of processed foods and the prevalence of corn oil, and experts agree that this imbalance can be a cause of heart disease and other health conditions.

If you're a vegetarian and you don't eat fish, flaxseed is a useful alternative. It's not as rich in Omega-3 EFAs as oily fish, but it really does help.

I have some delicious recipes using oily fish in the second part of this book, so you might like to give them a try: Salmon, Fennel and Quinoa Parcels (page 184), Mackerel with Rice and Rainbow Stir-Fry (page 186), Pink Trout with Buttered Lettuce (page 189) or Salmon Fishcakes (page 193).

5 Outside: Nourish your body

Just like your face, your body will benefit hugely from regular loving care with pure plant oils. After a bath, enjoy massaging oils into your body. Try using different blends of oils, depending on your needs. I like to use grapeseed as a massage oil base, as it is one of the lightest, but you could also use peach kernel or almond oil. All oil blends should be stored in glass containers and kept in a cool, dark place. Use within a month of making. Another quick fix is to add a few drops of avocado or rosehip oil to your body cream, then massage it on to your skin. This gives your skin a beautifully radiant, red-carpet gleam.

Here are some of my favourite oil blends.

Nourishing Oil Blend

120ml grapeseed oil

2 vitamin E capsules

20ml argan or rosehip seed oil

10 drops rose or neroli essential oil

Mix the ingredients together (pierce the capsules to release the oil) in a screw-top glass jar or bottle, and shake well before use. Apply to clean, dry skin.

Stimulating Oil Blend

120ml grapeseed oil
1 vitamin E capsule
10 drops rosemary essential oil

5 drops orange essential oil
2 drops peppermint essential oil

Mix the ingredients together (pierce the capsules to release the oil) in a screw-top glass jar or bottle, and shake well before use. Apply to clean, dry skin, concentrating on any areas of tension or sore, aching muscles.

Anti-cellulite Hip and Thigh Oil Blend

120ml grapeseed oil
1 vitamin E capsule

10 drops juniper essential oil
5 drops each lemon and fennel essential oil

Mix the oils together in a screw-top jar or bottle (pierce the capsules to release the oil) and shake well before use. Use daily on your bottom, hips and thighs, massaging well using firm circular movements. Not a miracle cure, but helpful for stimulating the circulation in this area.

HOW TO GIVE YOURSELF A BODY MASSAGE

- Pour a little oil into the palm of your hand and warm it gently by rubbing your hands together. Using long, sweeping strokes, massage the oil into your legs and arms – always working towards your heart. When you get to your knees and elbows, give them some special attention with small, firm, circular movements.

- Work up over your tummy and chest in gentle circular movements. When you get to your breasts, massage around each breast towards the armpit in an upward movement, then around the breast itself.

- Take a little more oil if you need to and cup your hands to pinch, knead and massage your neck. Start at the bottom of your neck, where it meets your shoulders, and work around the sides and up to base of the scalp. Stop at any sore spots and work with your fingers to ease any tightness.

- Rotate your shoulders forwards, then backwards a few times, then shake your arms to relieve any tension.

- Put a little more oil on the palms of your hands and sweep them up the front of your neck, finishing with a good massage along the jaw line and ending at the ears.

⑥ Inside: Eat nuts and seeds to nourish your skin

I love nuts and seeds – not only are they amazingly nutritious, they're also so convenient. I always carry some with me for when blood sugar levels dip, so I'm not tempted to grab a less healthy snack. Nuts and seeds are packed with protein, essential fatty acids, vitamins and minerals, and they're high in fibre, too. They're really skin-friendly as they contain lots of vitamin E, which helps keep our skin glowing and youthfully radiant.

These foods are great just as they are, but here are some other easy ways of making sure you include them in your daily diet.

- Blitz some almonds, walnuts, and sunflower and pumpkin seeds in a food processor and sprinkle them over yoghurt or porridge at breakfast time.

- Add a few chopped almonds, walnuts, pine nuts or pistachios to your salad. Or toast pumpkin seeds and add them as a garnish to salads or soups.

- For a healthy snack, spread an oatcake or rye toast with nut butter. You can make your own nut butters really easily – see page 221 for my recipes.

- Make your own nut-rich energy bars for a nourishing afternoon pick-me-up – see my recipe on page 119. Or try my Berry and Seed Beauty Bombs on page 132, which contain pumpkin, sunflower and sesame seeds for a tasty skin-friendly treat.

- Dress your salads with Pumpkin-Seed Dressing – nourishing and tasty (page 236).

- Enjoy a nut loaf for supper. My recipe on page 148 contains plenty of almonds and Brazil nuts.

- Mix yourself a pot of nuts and seeds, and keep some in your handbag or on your desk for a quick energy boost whenever you need it.

- A small handful of almonds in their skins make a skin-saving snack.

Soaking nuts

Generally speaking, I eat nuts and seeds without soaking them, but you can make them more digestible by doing this. Soaking neutralises the substances in them that prevent them germinating before conditions are right. These enzyme inhibitors are thought to put a strain on our digestive system and make it harder for us to benefit from all their amazing nutrients. Soaking nuts or seeds mimics what happens naturally when they are soaked by the rain, then start to germinate.

To soak almonds or hazelnuts, place them in a bowl of filtered room-temperature water with ½ tsp salt and leave them for 8–12 hours. After soaking, rinse the nuts well and leave them to air dry before eating them. Cashews and walnuts need only be soaked for about 4 hours, and pumpkin and sunflower seeds for about 8 hours. You can speed up the drying process by placing them in a very low oven for a few hours to dry, but take care not to roast them as this destroys much of their natural goodness.

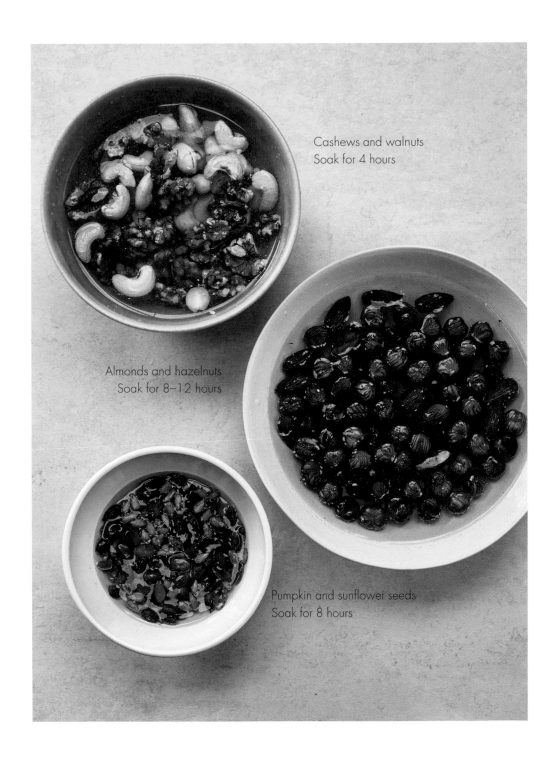

Cashews and walnuts
Soak for 4 hours

Almonds and hazelnuts
Soak for 8–12 hours

Pumpkin and sunflower seeds
Soak for 8 hours

⑦ Outside: Treat your hands and feet

Many of us lavish attention on our face but forget our hands and feet. They deserve our loving care too, especially as they often work so hard. However silky our cheeks, it is hard to look well groomed if our hands are rough-skinned and neglected – and any discomfort in our feet will soon show on our face. It's nice to treat yourself to a salon pedicure and manicure to keep your feet and hands in tip-top condition, but I enjoy giving myself a foot treatment at home too.

HOME PEDICURE

- First remove any nail varnish with an acetone-free remover, and soak your feet in a bowl of warm water for 5–10 minutes. If you have any kind of fungal infection, add a little tea tree oil to the water. Use a nail brush to give toenails a good scrub, and a foot file to help get rid of dry skin. If you like, add some marbles to the bowl and roll your feet over them to massage the soles.

- Dry your feet carefully, paying particular attention between your toes (dampness here can lead to infections such as athlete's foot). Trim your nails, cutting straight across them with scissors or clippers, then smooth the edges with an emery board.

- Rub a dab of cuticle cream or plant oil into your nails. Use a rubber hoof stick or wooden orange stick to gently push back the cuticles. Trim the hardened cuticle excess with cuticle nippers, taking care not to nick the skin.

- Give your feet a good massage with some body cream or special foot cream and rub a little oil into your toenails to nourish them (whatever you have handy). If you're doing your pedicure at night, slip on some cotton socks and leave the cream and oils to soak in overnight.

Cleansing Foot Scrub

75g coconut oil
25g Fuller's earth (from a chemist)
50g polenta

15 drops lemon, orange, peppermint or lavender essential oil

Melt the coconut oil and mix in the Fuller's earth to form a smooth paste. Add the polenta and essential oils of your choice, mixing well. Massage into clean, dry feet, focusing on the heels and calloused areas. Rinse well, patting the skin dry, and follow with a foot or body cream.

Our hands work hard. They're exposed to sun, wind and cold, constantly dipping in and out of washing-up water, and dealing with paper, detergents, cleaning products and so on. So once a week, try to give your hands some special care to keep them looking good.

- Start by washing your hands well in warm soapy water and giving your nails a good scrub. If your hands are particularly dirty – after gardening, for example – rub them with a cut lemon sprinkled with salt, or use a home-made hand scrub (see below).

- Remove nail polish with an acetone-free remover. Trim nails with nail scissors or clippers, and smooth them with a natural emery board or glass file (not metal). Always file in one direction rather than sawing back and forth. After filing, rinse your fingers in warm water and pat them dry.

- Put a little cuticle cream or oil (almond, avocado or grapeseed) on the nails and massage it into the cuticles. Leave for a few moments, then gently push the cuticles back with a rubber hoof stick or an orange stick wrapped with a little cotton wool.

- Put a generous dollop of hand cream on your hands and massage it in well, working all over your hands and up to your wrists and lower arms. Rub your knuckles well, massaging and pulling them to relieve stiffness. Take your time and enjoy this – it can be very relaxing.

- If you want to apply nail varnish, wipe away any remaining oil or cream residues from your nails first. Or simply add a little more oil to your nails to give them a lovely healthy shine, then buff with a nail buffer or soft cotton cloth.

Sugar Hand Scrub

Simply mix equal parts of granulated sugar with a good-quality cooking oil, such as rapeseed or olive oil (not extra virgin, as this is too thick and sticky). Add a drop or two of your favourite essential oil to give it a fragrance. Use on clean dry hands, scrubbing over the backs of the hands and around the cuticles, thumbs and wrists. Rinse well under warm running water and pat dry to leave the hands super-soft and exceptionally smooth.

WEEK FIVE:
Balance

We've looked at cleansing, healing and nourishing our skin, so now it's time to think about restoring our balance. Nothing makes our skin glow more than a true sense of calm, contented serenity. Balancing our foods helps too, so this is a good time to focus on potent plant oils, the natural ones found in nuts as well as my take on classic recipes made without gluten or dairy.

Try my Breakfast in a Glass recipe (page 99) enriched with rapeseed and multi-seeds, as well as some delicious and versatile Nut Butters (page 121). I'm also a big fan of making pies and quiche without pastry – such as my Broccoli and Feta Crustless Quiche (page 144) for better skin balance.

① Inside: Make sure you have your beauty sleep

My mother always said that one hour of sleep before midnight was worth two after midnight. As a teenager I didn't believe her, but now I know it's true! Too many late nights show in our face and our skin suffers. We do need our beauty sleep in order to stay looking good – it's not a myth. Research carried out at the Skin Study Centre in the United States concluded that those who slept badly had more wrinkles and slacker skin than good sleepers, and their skin lost water faster.

While we sleep, the body has a chance to repair itself – and that includes our skin cells – so a good night's sleep is essential for radiant skin. But I know all too well that it's not always easy to get the sleep I need, and so I've developed my own tried-and-tested night-time strategies.

Calm and comfortable
Try to keep your bedroom as a haven of peace. Ban phones, laptops and televisions, and if you want entertainment, read a printed book or listen to music. Electronic devices create electromagnetic radiation, which disrupts sleep patterns, and the light from screens also affects the pineal gland in our brain, causing it to produce less melatonin, the hormone that helps us sleep.

Ensure that your bed is as inviting as possible. Buy the best mattress you can afford and good supportive pillows. Don't forget to turn your mattress regularly (alternate upside-down and then side-to-side to prevent saggy spots), and experts advise replacing mattresses every 10 years. Mattress toppers add a lovely touch of luxury, as do good cotton sheets and duvet covers – such as those with a 400 thread count, or more. Some swear by silk pillowcases, saying they love the smooth feeling against their skin and that they don't wake with creased, crumpled cheeks.

Keep your bedroom as dark as you can with thick curtains or blinds. Some find sleep masks useful, especially when travelling. Avoid light-emitting alarm clocks or security sensors – put something over them, if necessary. I travel with a roll of black duct tape to screen off lights from hotel bedroom gadgets that pierce the darkness. Ideally your bedroom shouldn't be too warm. Best to have a lovely warm bed and a reasonably cool room – 15–20°C is about right.

MY TIPS FOR SOUND SLEEP

- It's clinically proven that we sleep better if we're not only active during the day and have some exercise, but also spend some time outside, in daylight. Experiencing that light/dark contrast helps us sleep.

- Stop having coffee, tea and dark chocolate (high in caffeine) six hours before your bedtime. So if you turn in at 11pm, have your last bit of caffeine at 5pm. I do enjoy a glass of wine in the evening, but too much alcohol can also disturb sleep.

- Eat your evening meal at least 2–3 hours before bedtime. A late, heavy meal can make it hard to sleep – and there's nothing like indigestion to keep you awake.

- We all know that babies and toddlers respond well to a bedtime routine, but so do grown-ups. It doesn't help if you're rushing around all evening before dropping into bed exhausted. Instead, adopt a gentle winding-down routine before bedtime, whether it's a soothing bath, listening to music, reading a book or magazine, or just pottering around putting clothes out for the morning.

- If you're feeling stressed about the next day, make a list of what you need to do. That way you're less likely to wake up at 3am fretting.

- If possible, keep your bedroom as quiet as possible. If there's a lot of outside noise – or if you have a partner who snores – try wearing earplugs.

- If you have trouble getting off to sleep, try putting a few drops of lavender oil on a cotton wool pad and popping it under your pillow. Inhale the soothing scent and it will help you drift off to sleep.

- If sleep doesn't come, don't try too hard. It will simply make you feel stressed. Enjoy the rest and relaxation and think about keeping your eyes open. It might seem odd, but sometimes just doing that can make you fall asleep.

- Try visualisation. Imagine a beautiful glow at the centre of your body. Then visualise that glow spreading out to your legs and feet, into your arms and up into your neck and shoulders, relaxing each part of the body as you do so.

And waking up ...

There's nothing worse than having to hurtle out of bed the moment you open your eyes. Allow yourself a few minutes to come to and stretch before you calmly rise and start your day. Also, waking to the jangle of an alarm is not pleasant. Consider buying a clock that wakes you more gently with a gradually brightening light instead of a loud noise.

② Outside: Take special care of your eyes

Our health shows in our eyes. When we're feeling well, our eyes are bright and sparkling. When we're tired or out of sorts, our eyes may appear red, dull or puffy, with dark circles or bags under them. In fact, dark circles aren't caused by tiredness but by fluid retention or a blocked nose. Both cause the veins under the eyes to become dilated, resulting in the appearance of dark circles. However, these dark circles can also be linked to health issues such as liver and kidney problems or thyroid disease; if they persist or are severe, do check with your doctor.

The skin around our eyes is particularly delicate and sensitive and is often the first place to show fine lines, so it deserves extra-special attention. Be careful not to drag or pull the skin when removing eye make-up. Moisturise very gently around your eyes, using a special eye cream if you like – look for one containing plant-based ingredients.

Sun damage

As it's so delicate, the skin around the eyes is easily damaged by sunlight. Apply a mineral-based sunscreen to your skin and wear sunglasses to protect your eyes in strong sun. Using concealer also adds a layer of helpful sun protection under the eyes.

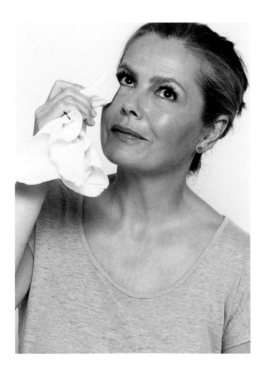

- Fill your washbasin with cold water and add some ice cubes. Splash the icy water over your eyes as many as 20 times if you can bear it, then pat them dry. This will reduce puffiness, clear redness and improve skin tone around the eyes. It's really refreshing, too. Alternatively, put some ice cubes in a muslin cloth and dab them around your eyes.

- Pop a couple of teaspoons in the fridge to chill for a while, then use them to gently massage around the eye area. This helps to ease fluid retention and refresh the eyes.

- Finely chop a little chilled cucumber and squeeze the juicy pulp on to a muslin cloth, lie down and place over your eyes for 10 minutes to soothe and brighten eyes. Or place used, squeezed-out camomile tea bags, chilled cucumber slices or raw potato slices on your eyes. All will help to tighten and freshen the delicate skin around the eyes. Used tea bags are also useful as they're full of natural tannins that can temporarily tighten skin. A good upcycling beauty tip!

③ Inside: Learn how to breathe properly

We don't need to think about breathing. We do it automatically, all the time – or do we? Yes, we have to keep breathing to live, but when we're busy and stressed our breathing can become shallow. We don't take in enough oxygen and that can contribute to our feeling tense and tired, which soon shows in our face. Breathing should be the easiest thing in the world, but it's worth taking some time out to become aware of it and breathe more effectively.

Think about what happens when we breathe. When we take a breath in, our diaphragm moves down so our lungs can expand. We take air in through our mouth or nose and down through the windpipe to the lungs. From there it passes through blood vessels to the heart, which pumps the oxygenated blood to every part of the body. The deeper the breath, the more air – and oxygen – we take in to nourish and revitalise our body.

In Eastern medicine, good breathing is considered essential to carry our essential life force, or qi, around the body. Only when the qi (pronounced 'chee') is flowing properly can our body be balanced and healthy – and that includes our skin.

Unfortunately too many of us sit in a hunched position, with our shoulders up around our ears and our body tight with tension; it's hard to breathe effectively that way. Whenever you feel particularly stressed and tired, stop and take some healing breaths. The world will be able to manage without you for 5 minutes – and you'll feel so much better for it.

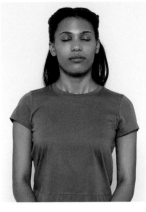 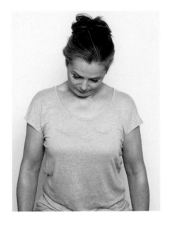 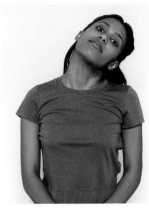

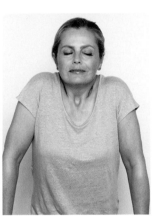 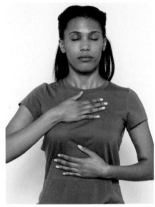 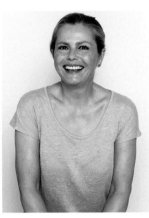

- Stand up straight with your weight evenly balanced on both feet, or sit comfortably but upright, feet flat on the floor. Shrug your shoulders right up, then sink them down again, as far as you can. Do this several times. Imagine that the top of your head is reaching up to the ceiling and try to release any tension in your neck. Very gently roll your head around a few times in each direction.

- Start taking deep, even breaths. Breathe in to a count of four or five, hold the breath for a couple of counts, then breathe out to a count of six. Keep your breathing as slow and steady as you can, and see if you can start breathing out to a count of seven or eight to really expel all the air from your body. Take the breath deep down to your abdomen when you breathe in.

- Close your eyes and imagine that life-giving breath extending to all corners of your body. Picture it flowing into your toes and fingertips, around your back and shoulders, and into your head.

- Focus on the feeling of your chest expanding and falling as you breathe in and out, but don't force it – let it happen naturally and gently.

④ Outside: Use the power of smell

I believe that we underestimate the importance of smell as a mood-enhancer and a way to improve our wellbeing. Nature has so much to offer in the form of essential oils, which not only smell glorious but can also have huge benefits for our skin and overall health.

Essential oils are indeed the very 'essence' of a plant, often described as its life force. They come from tiny oil glands present in most plants, and each has its own aroma and characteristics. Their use for beauty and health is not a modern fad. The Ancient Egyptians used perfumed oils, as did the Babylonians, Romans and others throughout the ages, but it was not until the twentieth century that their benefits were analysed scientifically and the term aromatherapy began to be used to describe a form of healing and therapy using essential oils.

Essential oils are quite different from edible oils, and are not meant for eating. Vegetable or plant cooking oils pressed from nuts and seeds are scientifically known as 'fixed' oils, whereas essential oils produced by distillation or solvent extraction are the fragrant 'volatile' oils. They can be used in a wide range of ways, from room-scenting vaporisers to massage blends, but adding them to a bath is one of the easiest and most delightful ways to enjoy them.

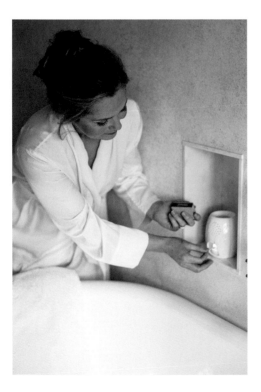

AROMA BATH

Run a bath, which should be warm rather than hot, as the oils are quickly broken down by heat. Once the bath is ready, dim the lights and close the bathroom door so the aromas don't escape.

Add the oil – just one kind, or a mixture of up to four. For adults, use up to eight drops of oil all together and stir them into the water well. Then step into the bath, lie back and relax. Breathe deeply and appreciate the soothing aromas.

AROMA SHOWER

If you don't have time for a bath, try an aroma shower. Wash yourself first, then add a few drops of essential oil to your sponge or flannel and rub it over your body while under the shower. Keep breathing deeply to inhale the scented vapours.

Bergamot – a wonderful aroma that can help relax and lift your mood.

Cedarwood – for soothing aching muscles and toning the skin.

Camomile – encourages sleep and for soothes irritated skin.

Geranium – for soothing skin.

Ginger – powerful and spicy. Good with citrus oils for a stimulating bath.

Jasmine – one of the most beautiful of all fragrances, and wonderful in the bath.

Lavender – aromatic, antiseptic, soothing, relaxing and healing.

Lemon balm – good for relieving tension when you need to relax.

Mandarin – has an uplifting and toning effect on the skin.

Marjoram – helps promote better sleep.

Neroli – a glorious scent, and makes a luxurious, cheering bath.

Patchouli – for a sensual and exotically aromatic bath.

Rose – expensive, luxurious and good for sensitive skin.

Rosemary – a stimulating pick-me-up.

Tea tree – cleansing and purifying. Use in tiny quantities.

Ylang-ylang – reviving, and helps lift the spirits.

Brilliant Bath Oil Blends

I have provided a few of my favourite oil blends on the page opposite. Add each of the oils to a pre-run bath, warm – not hot – for best effect. Swish around with your hands to disperse the scents before stepping in, and enjoy a soak for 10–15 minutes, topping up with hot water as required.

Scents as Pick-me-ups

Adding fragrance to our surroundings doesn't directly affect the skin, but can improve our mood and help put a smile on our face. I find I look better when I'm calm and relaxed too, so anything that helps here is useful. Essential oils are perfect for scenting our home, and so much better than commercial synthetic so-called air fresheners.

One method is to use a little oil burner that's heated with a night-light candle. You fill the top half of the burner with water, add a few drops of essential oil, then light the candle underneath. You do have to keep a careful eye on these though, as the water soon evaporates and the oil can burn. Simpler and safer is an electric oil burner – simply plug it in, add the oil to the padded applicator and the scent is gently diffused.

I also like the reed diffuser sets you can buy now, as these release a constant subtle aroma and need little attention. They're easy to re-fill yourself with your own choice of oil. I keep a small bottle of mixed neroli and lavender oils (two of my favourites) to top up my shop-bought reed diffusers at home.

Sensual and euphoric

Some essential oils are reputed aphrodisiacs – try this heady combination of exotic essences to get you in the mood …

4 drops patchouli   4 drops rose or
                             tuberose

Relaxing, for better sleep

Bath-time bliss for a better night's beauty sleep.

5 drops lavender
3 drops camomile

Tonic, for re-balancing mind and body

Calming and rejuvenating, this is an excellent duo for reviving both skin and psyche.

4 drops lemon balm   4 drops lavender
  or clary sage

Uplifting, to re-energise

Stimulating and refreshing, this is a great combo to give the body a bit of get-up-and-go!

4 drops rosemary,   4 drops ylang-ylang
  thyme or
  eucalyptus

Soothing and softening, for dry skin

Calming and nourishing, the ideal potion for parched skins.

5 drops camomile and 3 drops neroli, rose or geranium mixed in 1 teaspoon pure plant oil, such as almond, sunflower or peach kernel

⑤ Outside: Give yourself a reflexology foot massage to help rebalance the body

Reflexology is a fascinating complementary therapy and one that I believe really works. The theory is that all parts of the body are represented in the feet and are linked to reflex areas in the body. So by massaging and applying pressure to particular areas of the feet, you can ease different ailments.

Reflexology for the diagnosis or treatment of specific conditions should be carried out by a qualified practitioner, but you can enjoy massaging your own feet and relieving tension. It's nice to start by giving your feet a nice relaxing soak, then patting them dry. You can also give yourself a foot massage at home – see page 74 for more detail on how to do this.

- Support one foot on the opposite knee. Take some body oil or almond or olive oil and start massaging, beginning with the inner sole. There are many reflex points in this area, so you may come across sore spots. If you do, press and hold them gently and take a deep breath in and out.

- Continue massaging. If you feel tense or headachy, press the top of each toe with your thumbs and hold for 5–10 seconds while breathing deeply. The big toe is said to represent the head, with the base of the big toe corresponding to the neck. I find that working around the big toe with the thumb and forefinger, massaging any sore spots, can really help ease neck tension and headaches.

- To give your whole system a boost, use your thumb to follow a line from your second toe down to the centre of your foot. This area is said to relate to the solar plexus, the centre of our energy and emotions. Press this area firmly with your thumb for 5–10 seconds, while breathing deeply.

- To relax your back, use your thumb to massage along the inside arch of your foot in little circles. Start at the heel and work up to your big toe. This area corresponds with your spine, so if you come across any sore spots press for 5 seconds in that area. It's quite remarkable what you might find.

- Repeat on the other foot.

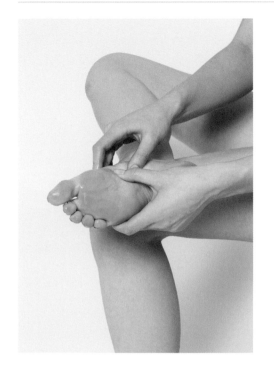

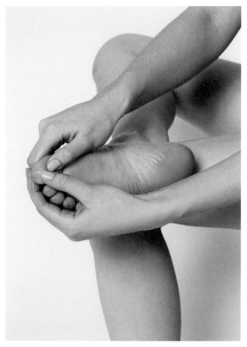

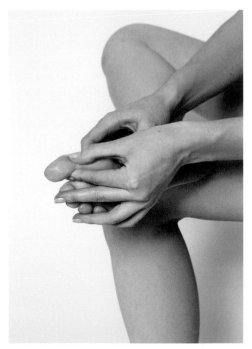

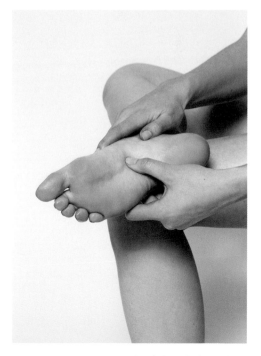

⑥ Inside: Try following the food combining diet

Some swear by food combining, not only as a way of losing weight, but also for better digestive balance and energy. At its most basic, food combining means not eating foods that 'fight' at the same meal.

It's an idea that was first developed back in the 1920s by Dr William Hay to treat his own health problems. His theory is that protein and carbohydrate are difficult to digest together, so by separating them and eating them at different meals the body uses food more efficiently and the digestive system is less stressed. There's little hard scientific evidence to prove this but, in practice, many people discover that after a couple of weeks on a food-combining regime they notice weight loss, better energy levels and healthier-looking skin.

Dr Hay believed that food combining was of great benefit to patients suffering from conditions such as diabetes, arthritis and allergies. It can also be helpful with skin conditions such as cellulite, psoriasis and eczema. Like Dr Hay, I believe that some skin conditions are a sign that all is not well inside the body and that food combining, which can help us digest our food properly and reduce waste matter or toxins, can only help our skin.

HOW IT WORKS

The main rule of food combining is to not mix carbohydrates (such as grains, bread, cereal, potatoes and sugar) with proteins (such as meat, fish, eggs and cheese) and acid fruits (grapefruits, oranges, lemons, etc.). The following are the basic guidelines:

- Make sure that vegetables, salad and fruit form the bulk of your diet.

- Don't eat starches and sugars at the same meal as proteins and acid fruits. Meals should be either starch-based (such as a baked potato and salad) or protein-based (such as fish and green vegetables).

- Avoid processed and refined foods such as white flour, sugar and processed fats.

- Avoid refined carbohydrates and eat only wholegrains, such as wholemeal bread and pasta, or wholegrain brown rice.

- Eat protein, starches and fats in moderation.

- Every day have one wholly alkaline meal (such as fresh fruit), one protein meal and one carbohydrate meal.

- Ideally, leave a 4-hour gap between a starch-based meal and a protein-based meal.

- Try to have a day a month when you eat only one kind of fresh fruit, such as apples, pears, kiwi or grapes. This is a great way to 'detoxify' and give your digestive system a rest.

7 Inside: Stress relief – taking time out for yourself

Stress is bad for your skin. It can be a trigger for acne and for inflammatory skin conditions, so it makes sense that any techniques for reducing stress can help towards good skin. Sadly, we're all so busy these days that there's very little opportunity for 'me-time'. When was the last time you sat quietly doing nothing – not sending emails, not listening to the radio or checking your phone? A few moments of quiet meditation daily can give you that inner peace and will be of great benefit to your overall health and appearance.

The immediate reaction of many people to the idea of meditation is 'I can't do that.' But you can – meditation is not something to be good or bad at. It's simply a matter of doing it – allowing yourself a few moments of peace and silence in the day. You don't have to believe anything in particular, you don't have to make strange noises or wear anything special. Meditation is just a way of calming and balancing your body, and many claim it can help improve your circulation, boost your immune system and help your concentration and focus.

Look at the face of someone who is stressed and anxious. Then look at the face of someone who is relaxed and at peace with themselves and you will see the difference that such stress-reduction techniques can make. There are lots of stress relief courses, apps and other guidelines, but you can start with a very simple form of meditation and build on that.

- Set aside some time – if possible, morning and evening – and find a quiet place where you won't be disturbed. Switch off your phone!

- Sit comfortably, preferably in an upright chair with your back straight, as it's important for energy to be able to flow up and down your spine.

- Breathe quietly. Relax each part of your body in turn, beginning with your face and jaw, working down to your neck and shoulders and onwards. Visualise each part tensing and relaxing.

- Close your eyes if you like. Some people like to repeat a single word over and over. Others prefer to picture a colour or a landscape.

- When other thoughts break in – which they will, particularly at first – don't worry, just let them go again. It doesn't mean you've failed. I imagine thoughts drifting into my head as clouds and visualise simply batting them away.

- At first, you might find you've had enough after 5 minutes, and that's fine. Gently bring yourself back into the world – don't leap up off your chair. Aim to build up to 10–15 minutes if you can.

WEEK SIX:
Maintenance and Radiance

Congratulations! You're at week six of my super-skin programme and I just know you'll be feeling – and showing – the benefits. Hopefully, most of the things we've been doing are now second nature to you and will become regular habits for a lifetime of fabulous, glowingly radiant, healthy skin.

So stock up with plenty of skin-friendly foods, such as my Beetroot, Carrot and Apple Crackers (page 125) as well as a stash of healthy, sweet-tasting treats, including Blackberry, Hazelnut and Spelt Cake Bites (page 218). And last but not least, reward your skin-saving journey with a healthy hoard of Beauty Bombs (page 132) for a delicious, nutritious treat all year round.

① Outside: Use a facial serum

Facial serums are relative newcomers in skincare, but most beauty ranges now include them. They can be very effective, and are well worth adding to our regular routine, especially for the over-30s, but not everyone knows exactly what they do and how to use them.

A serum contains highly concentrated active ingredients to help hydrate, lift and firm your skin, giving it a fresher, healthier look. The container may look small compared to a pot of moisturiser but that's because the serum doesn't contain the things like thickeners and sunscreens that can bulk out a normal moisturiser. You only need to use a small amount of serum at a time and the surface layers of skin absorb it quickly and efficiently.

Serums almost always contain antioxidants and anti-inflammatories as well as hydrating and so-called anti-ageing ingredients, and some are made to target certain problems, such as fine lines, dark spots or enlarged pores. Some are specifically designed to be used at night, while others can be used night or morning. All types of skin can benefit from serums, including oilier skin types. Choose your serum carefully for your particular needs. Although many are expensive, there are some good budget versions, so learn to study the labels and shop around.

To use a serum, clean your skin as usual and pat dry. Put some serum on your clean hand – a pea-sized amount should be enough – and smooth it over your face with clean fingertips. Using your fingertips, gently press the serum into your skin. Leave a little time for the serum to be absorbed, then apply your normal moisturiser over the top as usual.

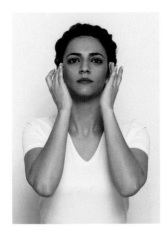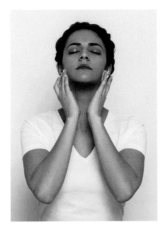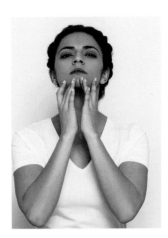
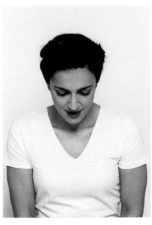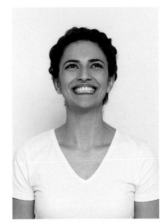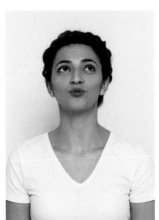

Facial exercises

We exercise the rest of our body, so why not our face? Facial exercises are not only good for strengthening saggy muscles, but moving our face helps boost blood flow, which in turn brings fresh nutrient-rich blood supplies to feed our complexion.

- To get the circulation going in your face, try tapping your skin. Using the pads of your middle fingers, tap out from the bridge of your nose along your eyebrows, then round and across the cheekbones. Tap up from the sides of your mouth, alongside your nose to the inner corners of your eyes. Then tap from your chin out along the jawline to each ear. Keep the taps very light and quick – you could also do this while applying your serum.

- Push your chin out and lift your bottom lip over your top lip. Hold it for a count of five. Repeat this ten times to help firm and tone your chin and neck.

- Say the words 'weeks' and 'queue'. Really exaggerate the words to widen and purse the lips. Repeat several times to exercise the muscles around your mouth.

② Inside: Keep up your aerobic exercise

Aerobic exercise (the kind that makes us out of breath) is vital for our general health and wellbeing. Cycling, running, jogging and going to the gym are all great for boosting our circulation and oxygenating the body – and they'll also bring a pleasing bloom to your skin. The official advice for adults is to have at least 150 minutes of moderate aerobic activity a week, as well as some core strengthening exercise, such as yoga, Pilates or weights, to work the muscles.

It's up to you how you take your exercise, but I believe that one of the easiest and most pleasurable ways is walking. It's free, you can do it anywhere, any time, and you don't need special equipment – other than a comfy pair of shoes. And research has shown that brisk walking is great for lifting the spirits and clearing the head. I find that when I get back to work after a good walk, my concentration is much improved and I'm full of ideas. That way you can take in your surroundings, appreciate nature and the ever-changing seasons, and enjoy being out in the light and air at the same time.

HERE ARE SOME GUIDELINES FOR GETTING THE MOST FROM YOUR WALKS

- Aim for at least 30 minutes most days of the week. If you want to lose weight, try doing 40 minutes, six days a week. You don't have to do your 30 or 40 minutes all in one chunk. If it's easier for you, break it up into a few walks of 10–15 minutes. You'll still get the benefit.

- Another good way of increasing your activity is to wear a simple pedometer, which measures the number of steps you do in a day. If you have a desk-bound job it can be quite alarming to see how low the number is if you don't put in a little extra effort. Aim to build up to 10,000 – or more – steps a day.

- For health benefits, walk briskly. If you feel your heart starting to pound and you're a bit out of breath but still able to hold a conversation, you're going at the right speed.

- Walk with your head held up, your shoulders relaxed and your back straight. As you walk, step forward with your heel first, rolling through to the ball of your foot and pushing off with your toes.

- When you've built up your stamina and you're in the habit of regular walks, you might like to up your fitness by trying power walking or Nordic walking. Power walking is simply walking at your maximum speed (4.5–5.5 miles an hour), which will increase your heart rate and consume more calories. For Nordic walking you walk with hand-held poles so that you're exercising your upper body at the same time as your lower body. It's fun, and great for fat-burning – and one of my all-time favourite exercises. You can even buy telescopic Nordic walking poles that pack away small for travelling.

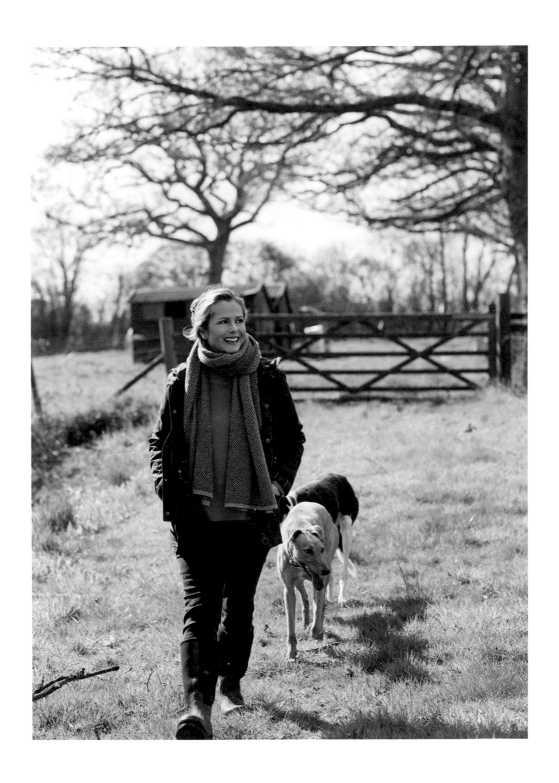

③ Outside: Look after your hair

The regime you've been following for your skin in terms of nutrient-rich foods and supplements will have done your hair a lot of good too, but it's worth also giving your crowning glory some special attention.

- Vitamin E, B complex vitamins and selenium are all great for hair health, and silica and zinc both help strengthen hair and nails. Green leafy vegetables, eggs, nuts and seeds are all good hair-friendly foods, as are olive oil and fish oils.

- Have your hair trimmed every 6–8 weeks to keep it in good condition and snip off any split ends.

- Avoid shampoos containing sodium lauryl/laureth sulphates. These are synthetic detergents that can aggravate dry, sensitive scalps – especially if you have any kind of sensitive skin condition, such as eczema or psoriasis. Instead, use plant-based shampoos with surfactants (often coming from corn or coconut derivatives), which can be much gentler on both your hair and scalp. It's amazing how often dandruff-type scalp disorders disappear when you make this simple switch.

- When washing your hair, don't use too much shampoo, which can strip away natural oils. Don't scrub too hard, which can over-stimulate the sebaceous glands, but just massage your scalp gently. One lather should be enough, unless you've been using lots of styling products. To create more lather, just add more water instead of more shampoo. One application of shampoo also makes any tinted or highlighted hair colours last twice as long as if you use two shampoos.

- Keep your use of hairspray and other styling products such as mousse and gels for special occasions only, as they can aggravate the scalp and leave a residue that soon builds up if used regularly. Using a styling mousse that doesn't touch the scalp is a better option than the more common liquid products if your scalp is very dry and sensitive.

- If you do have an itchy scalp, a simple paste made of baking soda can really help. Mix a spoonful of bicarbonate of soda with a little water to make a paste, and rub it on to your scalp after shampooing. Leave it for 10–15 minutes, then rinse off thoroughly. Another option is to rub some lemon juice or apple cider vinegar on to your scalp, leave it for 5–10 minutes, then rinse well.

- We all need to use conditioner, which protects the hair and gives it shine. Choose the right conditioner for your hair type and look for those containing plant oils, not silicones. If you have very fine hair, use a light conditioner and apply it only to the ends of the hair. If your hair is very dry or damaged by colour treatments, apply conditioner all over and leave it on for 5–10 minutes to penetrate the hair and work its magic.

- It's best not to use your hairdryer on the hottest setting, particularly if your hair is permed or coloured. Let your hair dry naturally as often as possible, or at least leave it until almost dry, then finish off with the hairdryer for final styling.

- Protect your hair from the sun – particularly if you have coloured or highlighted hair. Use a protective UV lotion or simply cover up with a hat or scarf in strong sun. To prevent fair or bleached hair from turning swimming-pool-green, always wet hair before plunging into a pool. This stops hair from soaking up so much of the chlorinated water that can give hair a greenish tinge.

Once a week or so, treat your hair to a nourishing overnight mask to bring back the gloss and shine. This is one of my favourites:

Glossy Hair Mask

50g coconut oil
50g cocoa butter
30ml almond or argan oil

15 drops of an essential oil of your choice
(neroli or lavender are some of my favourites)

In a small saucepan, simply melt the oils together, adding the essential oil last when all the others have melted and been removed from the heat. When the mixture is cool enough to touch, rub small amounts between the fingertips and apply sparingly to the hair, starting at the dry ends and working upwards. Keep any leftovers in a jar, and re-melt to use again. Wrap your head in a towel to help seal in body heat, or use a shower cap. Alternatively, sleep on a thickly folded towel to prevent the oils from staining your pillowcase. In the morning, apply your shampoo to dry hair before adding water (this makes the oils easier to remove). This occasional treat leaves even the driest locks with a glossy lustre.

4 Inside: Enjoy fresh fruit and vegetable juice every day

I am a huge fan of juicing. For me, it's not a fashionable fad but something I've been doing for 30 years or more, and that I've found enormously beneficial for my wellbeing as well as for my looks. Not only do fresh juices taste delicious, they're also an excellent way of increasing our intake of the skin-friendly vitamins and minerals that will keep us looking and feeling good. Juices give us an intense hit of nutrients – they're a perfect internal cleanser and a tonic to help give us clearer, more youthful-looking skin.

More and more we are learning that a poor diet contributes to many chronic illnesses. Fresh vegetable and fruit juices are brilliant for boosting health and vitality, so are great when you're recovering from illness, and they're a perfect way of getting extra nutrients into children and teenagers. For older people, juices are easy to digest and can be an excellent vitality boost.

And for everyone, juices are easy to make and a sheer pleasure to drink.

Juices are great for detoxing – I like to have a juice-only day or two once in a while – and they're also perfect when you're on a weight-loss regime. Juices are relatively low in calories (especially the low-sugar vegetable kind) and pretty much fat-free, but still satisfying, and so they help those hunger pangs. When you're dieting, be sure to use many more vegetables than fruit in your juices so you don't consume too much sugar.

You can of course buy juices, but it is far better to make your own. You know exactly what's in them for a start – some ready-made juices can contain additives and preservatives. Making your own also means you can tailor your juice to your own needs. Also, juice should ideally be consumed within a few hours of making to get the best of the nutrients. After that juices start to lose their fresh enzyme activity and some of their vitality.

HERE ARE SOME TIPS FOR HAPPY JUICING

Use raw ingredients, or organic if possible. If you can't buy organic fruit and vegetables, give them a good wash in warm water with a mild detergent, then rinse well, and dry.

Go for 70 per cent vegetables with 30 per cent fruit as a general rule, so you don't take in too much sugar. Fruit alone can cause a sugar rush, so be sure to mix the sweetest fruits such as grapes and pineapple with green veg for a better balance.

Don't glug your juice down in big gulps. Serve in small glasses and take your time to savour and sip it – try to 'chew' your juice to get your digestive enzymes flowing.

Variety is key – choose from a wide range of veg and fruit and go for different colours – dark green veg, purple berries, orange carrots – to be sure of getting different nutrients. The darker the colour, the more nutrients a piece of fruit or veg contains.

Juicers vs. blenders – which is best?
I generally use a juicer, which extracts the juice from fruit and vegetables and leaves the pulp. You can add some of this pulp to your juice if you like, but there tends to be quite a bit left over. I use this leftover pulp to make fantastically tasty crackers (see page 125), and it also makes great compost, so don't waste it. Powerful machines such as the NutriBullet, Vitamix or other blender-style kitchen gadgets blitz the whole fruit or vegetable into a more smoothie-type drink, thinned with water, so there is very little waste. Each system has its fans. Some prefer the fresher taste of the pure juice while others swear by the smoothie style. It's up to you – rest assured that whichever you choose you'll be doing your body a favour. See pages 245–246 for some of my favourite skin-friendly smoothies and fresh juices.

⑤ Outside: Give yourself a facial

I love a professional facial once in a while for a treat, but it's also fun to give myself a regular treatment at home. A home-style facial makes a real, visible difference to skin, too. I get everything ready in advance, switch off my phone and settle down for some blissful bathroom 'me-time'. Here's what to do:

- Cleanse your face thoroughly with a creamy cleanser, then remove the cleanser with a pure cotton cloth or a fine flannel wrung out in warm water.

- Exfoliate with a good (gentle) facial scrub or one you've made yourself (see page 19 for my recipes). This helps to get rid of dead skin cells and freshens the complexion. Avoid the eye area when applying exfoliators, but don't forget to pay attention to your neck and chest. Use any excess on the backs of your hands, too.

- Now it's time for a steam that will soften the skin and help to give a really deep cleanse. Fill a bowl with just-boiled water. Add a few drops of essential oil or a sprinkling of herbs (rosemary and lavender are two of my favourites), then lean over the bowl and put a large towel over your head and neck to form a tent. Breathe deeply for a few minutes, then remove the towel and pat your face dry. (See pages 34–35 for more information on this method.)

- Apply a face mask. There are plenty of good ones to buy, or you can make your own using my recipe on page 44. Smooth it over your face and neck, avoiding the eye area, lips and hairline. Lie back and relax for 10–15 minutes and let the mask do its work. You could also put some cucumber slices or squeezed-out tea bags over your eyes to soothe them at the same time. When you're ready, rinse the mask off and splash your face with cool water.

- Spray a little alcohol-free toner or pure rose water on to a cotton wool pad and wipe over your face to refresh your skin.

- Finally, moisturise. You could take this opportunity to apply your moisturiser extra-carefully, perhaps using some serum or facial oil first. Massage the oil or moisturiser in well, not forgetting your neck and chest.

- Go to bed, sleep well … and wake up looking radiant!

⑥ Inside: Superfoods

I like to make my daily fruit and vegetable juices even more nutritious and nurturing by adding some special extra ingredients. These are some of my favourite super-skin foods that you might like to try:

Chlorella is a type of green algae that grows in fresh water. It's available in tablet form but also as liquid extract or powder that you can add to juices and smoothies. It contains plenty of chlorophyll (plant protein) as well as vitamins, minerals (including absorbable iron, so it's ideal for vegans) and amino acids. I've found it to be very good for overall skin health. Not everyone, though, can tolerate chlorella so do check with your doctor if you have a chronic medical condition.

Spirulina is also a freshwater algae. It's a rich source of protein and is packed with vitamins B and E, minerals such as calcium and iron, and chlorophyll. It has a slightly milder taste than chlorella so it's easier to take in a breakfast juice or smoothie. Rich in plant protein, spirulina is every vegan's best friend.

Barley grass is a powder made from leaves, which are gathered young and dried. It's an excellent source of soluble dietary fibre, chlorophyll and magnesium, and is reputedly good for helping to alkalise the body. It is more easily absorbed than wheatgrass.

Wheatgrass also contains lots of nutrients and is one of the best sources of chlorophyll. It's available as a liquid or a powder made from young wheatgrass shoots, and contains vitamins such as beta-carotene, C, E and K as well as B-complex vitamins and minerals including iron, zinc, copper, manganese and selenium. Also helpful as a supplement for vegetarians and vegans, it's said to be both alkalising and helpful for supporting the immune system, as well as promoting glowing skin and shiny hair. If you like, you can also grow your own wheatgrass in your kitchen and snip the shoots straight into your juicer.

Hemp seeds are a good source of Omega-3 (also found in fish oils) as well as protein and minerals. They're available as a powder, so are very easy to add to juices or smoothies.

Herbs such as parsley, coriander and basil are not quite such powerhouses as wheatgrass and spirulina but they're an excellent flavourful addition to juices. Parsley, for example, is very rich in vitamin C.

Sprouted seeds and beans are easy to grow yourself and can be added to juice. You can grow shoots from seeds such as alfalfa on damp kitchen paper or in a special germinator tray. The sprouting action of these seeds and beans is said to trigger a powerhouse of active germinating enzymes that can also give our health and vitality a boost.

⑦ Outside: Great skin forever

I really hope that if you've enjoyed all my advice and tips in the previous pages over the last 6 weeks, your skin is looking smoother and more radiant than ever before – and that you're bursting with health and vitality! Do share your superb-skin selfies on Facebook, Instagram and Twitter – just tag me at Liz Earle Wellbeing or use #skinfoods. To keep your skin its radiant best, try to make these the healthy habits of a lifetime, not just for six weeks.

Please do your best not to go back to old eating habits and foods laden with synthetic additives and refined sugars. Stick to wholesome, traditional and unprocessed ingredients, with plenty of vegetables and some fruit – make sure you try the recipes in the second part of this book, and you won't go far wrong. Snack on my very delicious beauty bombs (see pages 132–133), nuts and seeds and a little dark chocolate instead of cakes and biscuits. Keep your fluid intake high with plenty of pure, filtered water sipped throughout the day, and by all means enjoy the odd cup of coffee or tea (and a glass of wine with supper in the evening) but try not to overdo it. If you're heading out to a party, keep in mind that clear spirits are the purest for the skin, so vodka mixed with a fresh juice is by far your best choice, with plenty of water alongside.

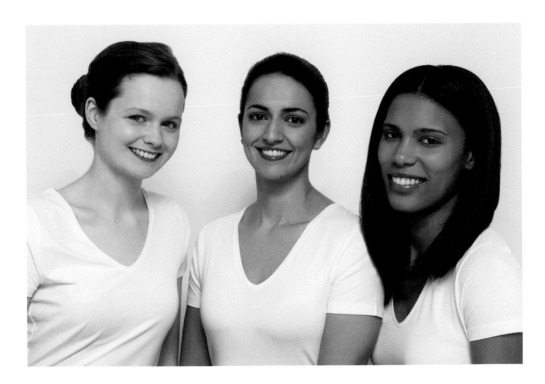

Every day:

- Cleanse your face with a foam-free cleanser twice a day, every day.

- Moisturise your face with a plant-oil based cream, twice a day, every day.

- Use a high-factor mineral-based sunscreen on your face, neck and backs of the hands when outside in the sunshine (and all over when the sun is strong).

- Drink plenty of filtered water – 1.5–2 litres sipped throughout the day.

- Eat unprocessed foods, with plenty of plant matter, green veggies and some fruit.

- Keep up the juicing – aim to have at least one mainly vegetable juice every day.

- Keep up the nutritional supplements – multivitamins, minerals and probiotics (such as acidophilus).

- Exercise – take a walk, do some stretches, stay active.

- Breathe – remind yourself to breathe properly and relax your shoulders to de-stress yourself.

- Be still – give yourself a few moments of quietness, meditation or prayer in the day to clear your head and calm your body.

- Dry-skin body brush, then enjoy a soothing aroma bath or aroma shower. Apply body cream after your bath or shower.

- Sleep for 7–8 hours every night.

Every week:

- Give yourself a facial or a facial steam.

- Apply a face mask.

- Enjoy a home manicure.

- Give yourself a body scrub.

Every fortnight:

- Enjoy a home pedicure with some added reflexology foot massage.

Every month:

- Consider having a juice- or one fruit-only day, e.g. apples.

- Book a beauty treatment, such as an all-over body massage or a professional facial.

Every 3 months:

- Consider a 48-hour inner cleanse.

And now … Let's Eat!

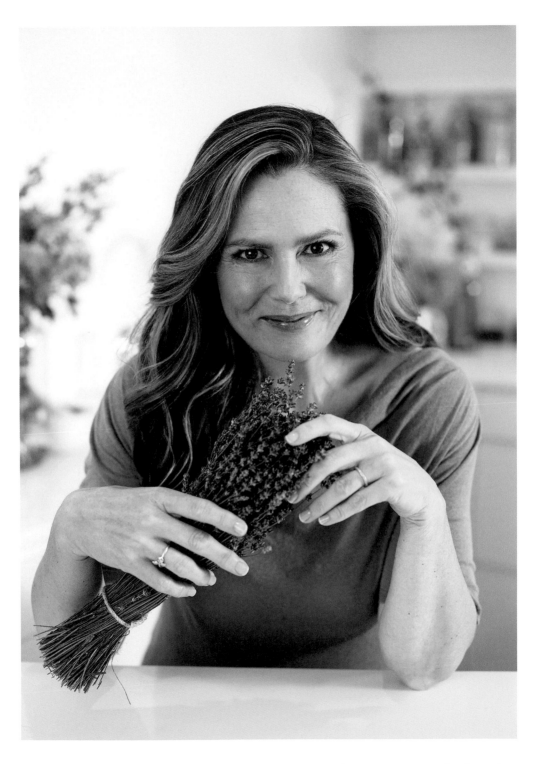

PART TWO: SKIN RECIPES

BREAKFAST

Cinnamon-toasted Oats with Yoghurt and Summer Fruit

This is a very quick breakfast and makes a lovely change from porridge. For extra flavour, I like to add a little ground ginger along with the cinnamon, but it's up to you. And you might even want to start making your own yoghurt – see my tip below. All you need to start is organic milk, some organic yoghurt and a digital thermometer to check the temperature along the way.

v SERVES 1   261 calories

25g jumbo oats

1 tsp mixed seeds, such as linseeds, poppy seeds, sunflower seeds, sesame seeds

½–1 tsp ground cinnamon

Good pinch ground ginger (optional)

100g summer fruits, such as strawberries, raspberries, blueberries

125g natural organic yoghurt

- Put the oats and seeds in a frying pan and toast over a medium heat for around 3 minutes, until the seeds start to pop. Toss the pan every now and then to ensure everything toasts evenly.

- Stir in the cinnamon and ginger, if using, and toss again. Cook for 1 minute more.

- Spoon the fruit into a large glass, top with the yoghurt, then spoon over the toasted oat mixture. There'll be a satisfying sizzle as the hot oats hit the cold yoghurt. Enjoy straight away.

LIZ'S TIP

Make your own yoghurt – it's very easy to do. Pour 600ml of milk into a saucepan and place over a medium heat. Heat until the temperature reaches around 80–85°C – just before it starts to boil. Remove the pan from the heat, cover with a lid and wrap the whole pan in a clean tea towel or two. Set it aside and keep checking the temperature every half hour until it drops to 45°C. Put 2 heaped tablespoons of natural organic yoghurt into a bowl, then stir in a couple of tablespoons of the milk. Return this yoghurt mixture to the pan. Cover with a lid, then wrap the pan in towels to keep the heat in and put it in a warm place, such as a just-turned-off oven. The mixture will set at around 43°C.

Transfer the mixture to a clean container, cover and chill. If the mixture has separated slightly, whisk it together to make a creamy yoghurt. Enjoy within 1 week.

When you've used almost all the yoghurt up, make another batch with the last 2 heaped tablespoons of this yoghurt, and start the process all over again.

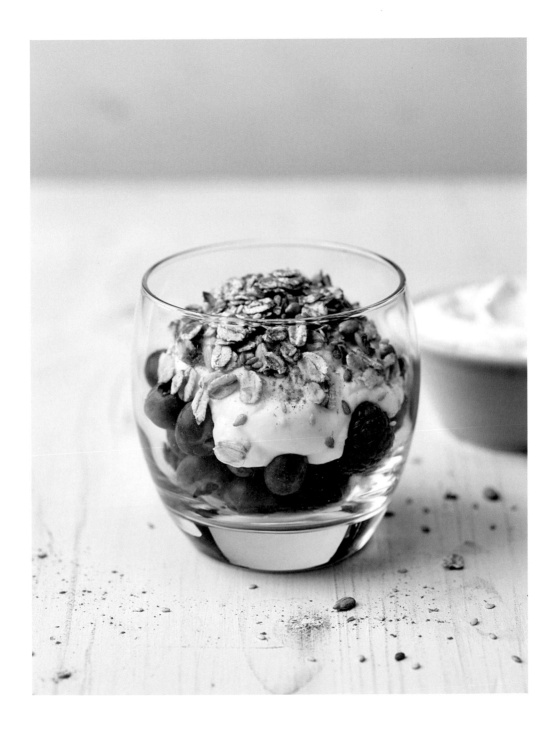

Home-made Muesli

This muesli is delicious with full-fat milk (I like to buy organic and pasture-fed whenever I can) and fresh fruit, or topped with a spoonful of yoghurt and a sprinkling of cinnamon. If you would like to ensure the recipe is dairy-free, use dairy-free milk or yoghurt. If you prefer less chunky muesli, put the jumbo oats into a food processor and whizz for 3–5 seconds to chop them roughly, then add them to the mix. I find it easier to put the muesli into a large shallow container so that I get a good selection of all the goodies in the mix.

 V DF   MAKES 20 PORTIONS, EACH 50G   210 calories

400g jumbo oats
125g barley flakes
125g buckwheat flakes
50g ready-to-eat dried dates, chopped
50g sultanas
50g dried unsweetened mango, chopped

50g whole almonds, chopped
50g hazelnuts
50g linseeds
25g sunflower seeds
25g pumpkin seeds

- Put the oats, barley and buckwheat in a large bowl, then add the dried fruit. Toss everything to combine, and make sure none of the fruit is sticking together.

- Add the nuts and seeds and give all the ingredients a good stir again. Spoon into a large shallow sealable container, and use within 1 month.

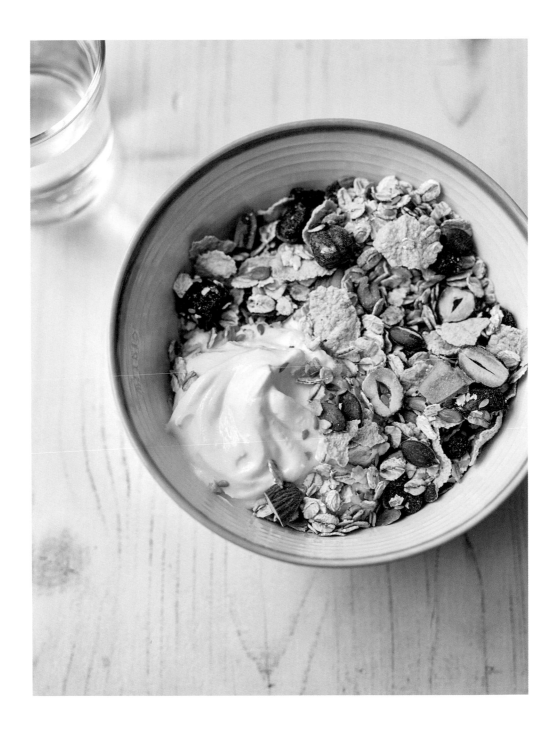

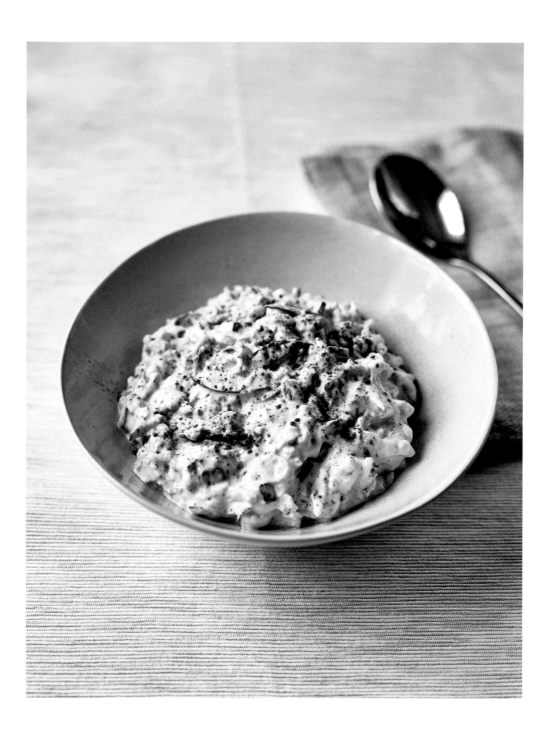

Liz's Bircher Breakfast

It's best to use jumbo rolled oats for this breakfast, otherwise the finished bircher can end up with a slightly mushy texture. I've added a tip below to help you make your own almond milk, too.

v   SERVES 1   387 calories

10g flaked almonds
10g pumpkin seeds
30g jumbo rolled oats
1 apple, cored and grated
50ml almond milk (see tip below to make
  your own)

100g home-made natural yoghurt (see page 92)
  or Greek yoghurt
Ground cinnamon, to serve

- The night before you want to serve the bircher, put the flaked almonds, pumpkin seeds, oats and apple into a small sealable container. Stir in the almond milk and leave overnight in the fridge.

- The next day, take the box out of the fridge and spoon the oat mixture into a bowl. Stir in the yoghurt and serve sprinkled with a little cinnamon.

LIZ'S TIP

Make your own almond milk. Put 50g of whole almonds in a bowl and add enough water to just cover the nuts (around 85g). Leave to soak for 4–6 hours, then drain well. Put the almonds and water in a food processor with 150ml of cold water and whizz until the nuts are finely ground and the water looks milky. Strain through a sieve into a bowl, pushing the mixture down with the back of a spoon to extract all the liquid. Use any leftover almond grains in the Tropical Energy Bars (see page 119) in place of the flaked almonds.

Alternatively, stir half of this almond grain and milk mixture together with the jumbo oats and grated apple (see quantities above) and leave overnight in the fridge. The next day, stir in the yoghurt and sprinkle with the cinnamon. Store the remaining milk and almond grains in the fridge for another breakfast.

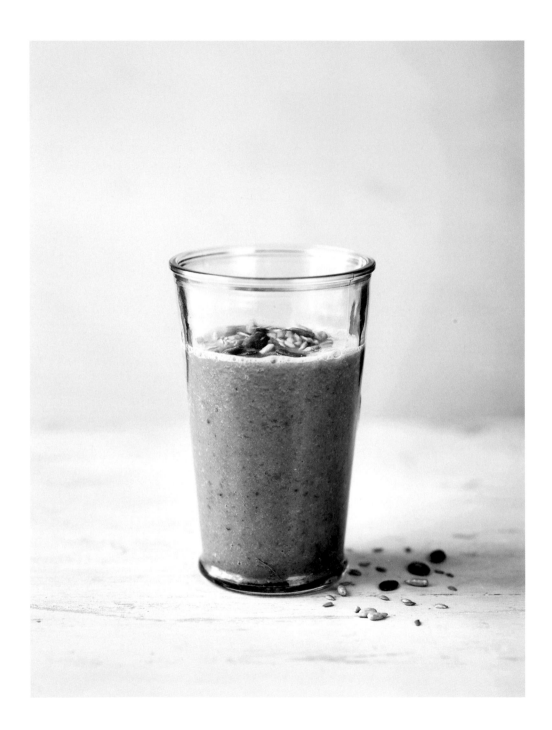

Liz's Breakfast in a Glass

I always feel as though my skin is being thoroughly nourished while sipping this! I've suggested two different apple varieties that I think work well here – my particular favourite is the russet, as it has such a nutty flavour. I love the crunchy seed topping and you could even splash a little Tabasco on top if you like.

 V DF GF SERVES 1   230 calories

½ banana, peeled
½ apple, such as Cox's or Egremont Russet
¼ avocado, peeled and stoned
50g spinach, washed
1 tsp rapeseed oil or olive oil
125–150ml cold water

For the topping:
½ tsp linseeds
1 tsp pumpkin seeds
1 tsp sunflower seeds

- Put all the seeds for the topping in a frying pan and place over a medium heat. Allow to cook for 2–3 minutes until golden, shaking the pan every now and then.

- Make the juice by blending the banana, apple, avocado, spinach and oil in a mini food processor until you have a smooth purée. Add the water and whizz again.

- Pour into a glass, top with the seeds and serve.

Poached Egg Nests

I love a protein-based breakfast, especially at the weekend when there's a bit more time. This is a firm family favourite.

GF SERVES 1   200 calories

1 medium or large egg, broken into a small bowl
100g spinach, washed
5g unsalted butter

Freshly grated nutmeg
30g good-quality smoked salmon
Sea salt and freshly ground black pepper

- Bring a small saucepan of water to the boil. Turn the heat down a little so it's simmering, and swirl the centre with a spoon. Carefully lower the egg into the middle and leave to poach for 3½–4 minutes, until the white has set but the yolk is still runny.

- Meanwhile, put the spinach in a separate saucepan with the butter. Cover with a lid, and wilt over a gentle heat. Season well with the nutmeg, salt and pepper.

- Arrange the wilted spinach in a round on a plate, then top with the smoked salmon. Tear up the pieces if they seem too big. Carefully drain the egg on kitchen paper and place in the middle of the salmon. Season with more nutmeg, and serve.

LIZ'S TIP

If you're cooking this for others too, this recipe is easy to multiply. For the eggs, though, you may find it easier to poach them in cling film so they can all cook at the same time. To do this, cut a small square of cling film, and brush it with olive oil. Push it into a ramekin and crack the egg into the cling film. Wrap the cling film tightly around the egg so there's no air, and twist to secure the ends. Do the same with the other eggs that you're cooking, and cook them all in the pan at the same time, as directed.

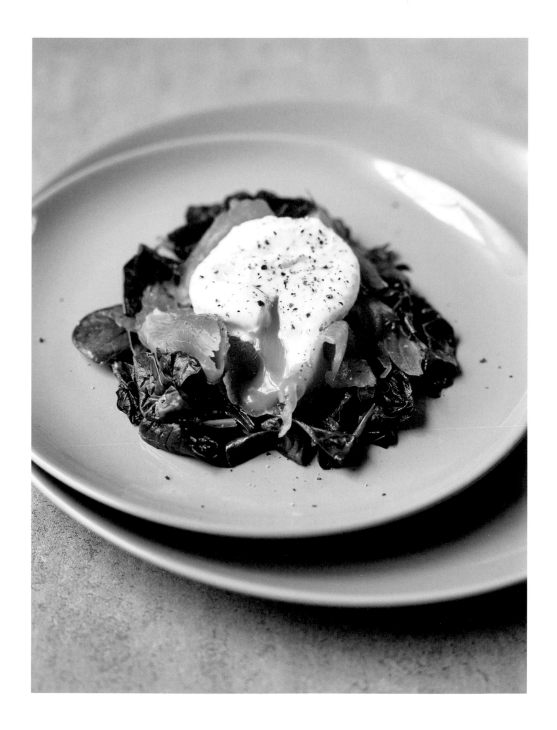

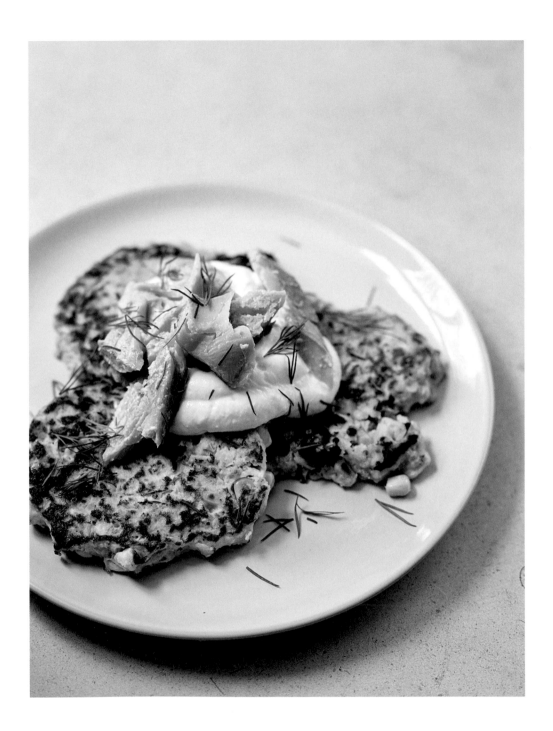

Courgette and Summer Corn Pancakes

We often have these pancakes for a weekend breakfast treat and my children enjoy helping to make them. They contain good carbs and some protein so they're really filling as well as delicious. Leave out the trout to ensure a vegetarian recipe.

v   SERVES 4   188 calories

100g ricotta
1 egg
50g oats, finely ground
1 small courgette (125g), grated
½ corn on the cob, kernels removed
1 tsp olive oil or flaxseed oil, for frying
Sea salt and freshly ground black pepper

To serve:
4 tbsp Greek yoghurt
125g smoked trout, cut into 4 pieces
A few sprigs dill, to garnish

- Fold the ricotta and egg together in a bowl and season well. Add the oats, courgette and corn kernels, and mix again. Set aside for 15 minutes to allow the oat flour to absorb the liquid.

- Heat the oil in a frying pan over a medium heat, until hot. Turn the heat down low. Use a dessertspoon to scoop up the pancake mixture and carefully place it in the pan. Repeat twice more so you're frying three pancakes at a time. Allow to cook for around 2 minutes, until golden, then flip over and cook for another 2–3 minutes. Set aside on a plate.

- Continue to cook the pancakes in batches of three, until all the mixture has been used up – you should have 12 pancakes in total.

- Divide the pancakes between four plates, top with a little Greek yoghurt and a piece of trout, and garnish with dill.

Banana, Oat and Nut Butter Pancakes

These are lovely and filling and the oats make them much firmer than American pancakes. It really is worth leaving the batter to stand for 10 minutes before using so the grains swell up – this makes the pancakes easier to handle and turn. With a spoonful of Greek yoghurt and some fruit, these make a very wholesome breakfast.

v   SERVES 4   186 calories

50g rolled oats, roughly ground
50g Smooth Almond and Cinnamon Butter or
    Chunky Peanut Butter (see page 121)
1 banana, peeled and roughly chopped
2 medium eggs
A little flaxseed oil, for frying

To serve:
Natural Greek yoghurt
Summer fruits, such as raspberries and blueberries

- Put the oats in a large bowl. Whizz the nut butter and banana together in a small blender, and add the mixture to the oats. Whisk in the eggs. Set aside for 10 minutes to allow the grains to absorb the liquid and swell.

- Put ½ teaspoon oil in a frying pan and heat over a medium heat until hot. Turn the heat down to low and use a teaspoon to scoop up some of the mixture and place it in the pan. Do the same twice more to make three small pancakes and cook for around 2 minutes until golden underneath. Flip over and cook on the other side until golden.

- Continue to cook the pancakes in batches until you've made around 12. Serve three per person, with a spoonful of Greek yoghurt and the summer fruit.

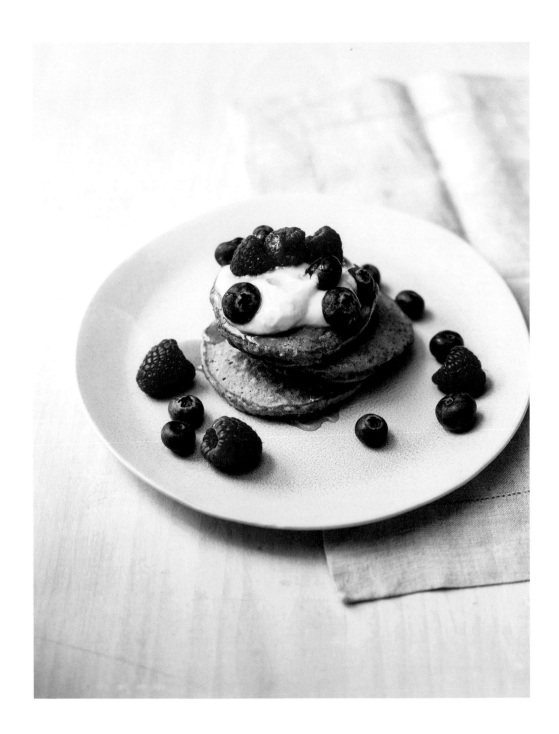

Basil, Cherry Tomato and Goat's Cheese Omelette

This omelette makes an excellent skin-friendly start to the day. It's bursting with high-quality protein and fats that are good for the skin – and it's so tasty, too.

V GF SERVES 1   292 calories

1 tsp olive or flaxseed oil
5 cherry tomatoes, halved
1 spring onion, finely sliced
2 medium eggs

1 tsp linseeds
3–4 basil leaves, torn into small pieces, plus extra
   to garnish
20g soft goat's cheese
Sea salt and freshly ground black pepper

- Heat the oil in a frying pan and sauté the cherry tomatoes and spring onion for 2–3 minutes, until golden.

- Beat the eggs in a bowl with the linseeds and seasoning. Add the basil to the eggs.

- Slowly pour this mixture into the pan, allowing the egg to run into the holes. Scrape a spatula along the edge of the set egg and pull it towards you across about a third of the pan. Tilt the pan again and allow the remaining egg to run into the empty space.

- Set the pan level on the hob again and cook the omelette for about 1 minute, until the top has set. Dot over the goat's cheese, then flip over one side of the omelette and fold the other side over the top. Slide the omelette on to a plate and serve with a few extra basil leaves.

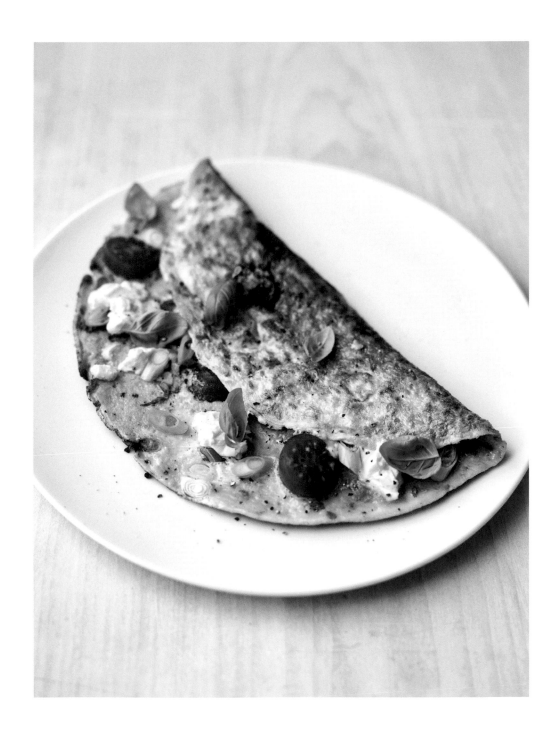

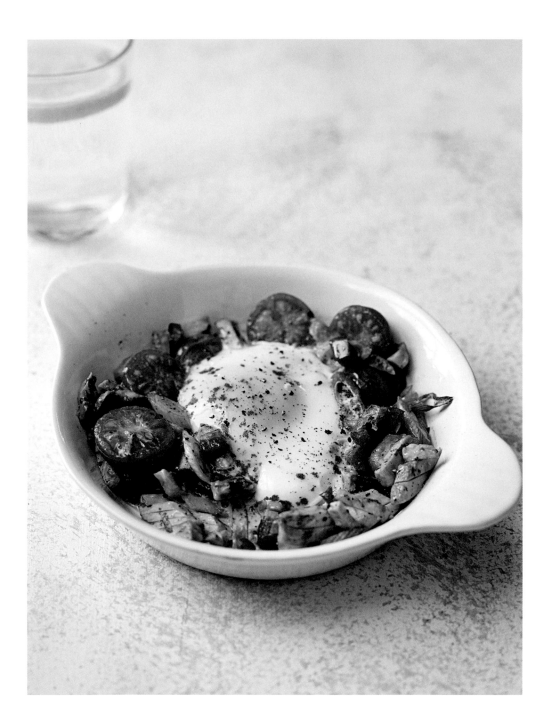

Baked Avocado Eggs

This is my twist on baked avocado and packs in a few more veggies. It's very easy – takes about 5 minutes to prepare, then the oven does all the hard work. The warm soft avocado and just tender vegetables make a perfect combination of textures and flavours.

V DF GF   SERVES 4   200 calories

1 avocado, peeled, stoned and chopped   1 tsp olive oil
16 cherry tomatoes, halved   Good pinch cayenne pepper
1 red pepper, halved, deseeded and chopped   4 large eggs
4 small spring onions, chopped   Sea salt and freshly ground black pepper
1 tbsp chopped fresh parsley

- Preheat the oven to 200°C/400°F/Gas mark 6.

- Put the avocado, tomato, red pepper, spring onions and parsley in a bowl. Add the olive oil and season well with the salt, pepper and cayenne. Toss everything together. Divide evenly between four shallow ovenproof dishes, trying to spoon an equal amount of each ingredient into each dish. The ingredients should form a single layer at the bottom.

- Make a well in the middle of each and crack the eggs into it, allowing the white to run into the vegetables. Bake in the oven for 15 minutes, until the eggs are set. Serve straight away.

LIZ'S TIP

If you're making this just for yourself, use the following quantities: ¼ avocado, 4 cherry tomatoes, ¼ deseeded red pepper, 1 spring onion, 1 teaspoon chopped fresh parsley, ¼ teaspoon olive oil, seasoning and a small pinch of the cayenne, and 1 large egg.

Kippers with a Crunch

My family just love kippers and I like to make this for breakfast or brunch in the holidays. Make sure you serve it with plenty of juicy fresh lemon wedges to squeeze over. It's good with smoked haddock, too if you're not a kipper fan.

SERVES 4   342 calories

2 kippers (or 2 smoked haddock fillets – each
    around 230g)
15g jumbo oats
1 tsp sunflower seeds
1 tsp pumpkin seeds
1 tsp linseeds
1 tsp flaxseed or olive oil
Freshly ground black pepper

To serve:
200g spinach, washed
20g unsalted butter
Freshly grated nutmeg
½ lemon, cut into 4 wedges
Freshly ground pepper

- Preheat the grill. Put the fish, skin-side down, on a baking sheet, and grill for 5 minutes.

- Stir together the oats, sunflower seeds, pumpkin seeds, linseeds and oil, and season with pepper. Scatter the mixture over the fish and continue to grill until the fish is cooked and the topping is just golden (this will take around 5 minutes). If you're cooking smoked haddock, you may need to cook the fillets for 2–3 minutes longer, depending on how thick they are.

- Put the spinach and butter into a large saucepan and cover with a lid. Place the pan over a high heat for 2–3 minutes until the spinach has wilted. Season with nutmeg and pepper. Spoon the wilted spinach on to four plates. Halve the fish pieces, and place each on top of the spinach. Serve with a lemon wedge to squeeze over.

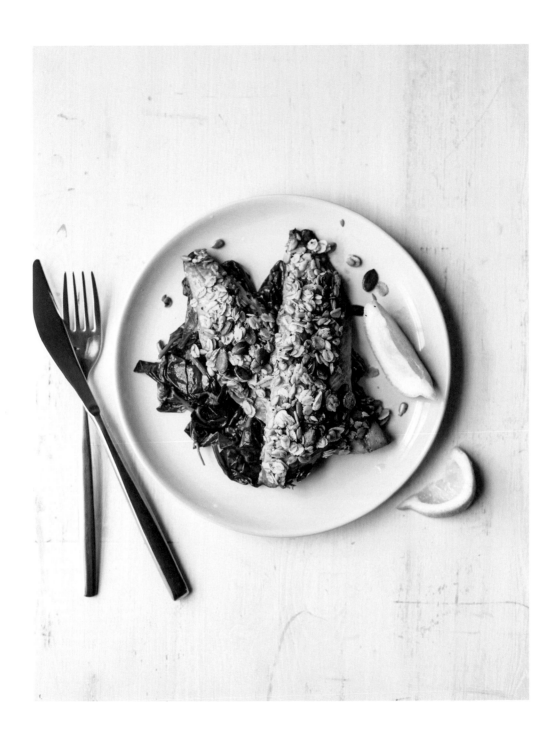

SKIN SNACKS

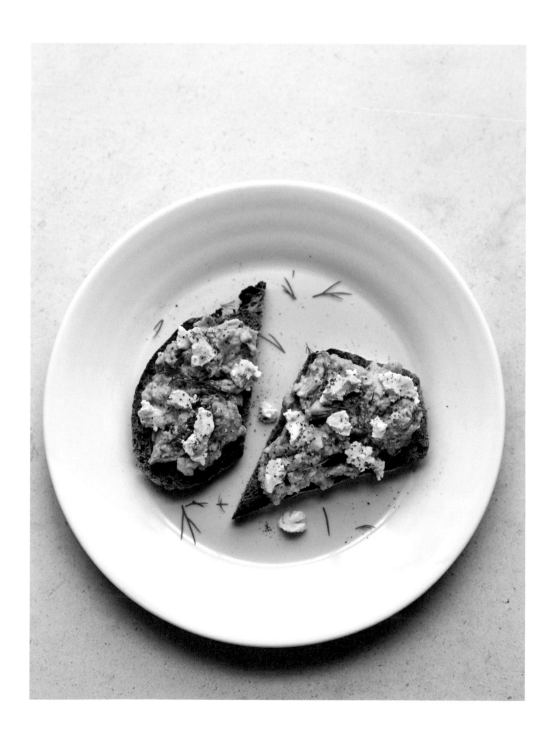

Avocado on Rye

Avocados are such a great skin food, whether you put them in or on your body. This classic is delicious, nutritious and very filling.

SERVES 1, OR MAKES 8 CANAPÉ SQUARES   300 calories

1 slice dark rye bread
½ avocado, stoned
Zest and juice of ¼ lime
Good pinch smoked paprika
2 sprigs dill, plus an extra sprig to garnish

50g smoked trout, roughly broken up, or soft
   goat's cheese, chopped or crumbled into
   small pieces
Sea salt and freshly ground black pepper

- Toast the rye bread on both sides.

- Scoop the avocado flesh out of the skin and put it in a bowl. Add the lime zest and juice, smoked paprika and seasoning. Snip the dill over the top, then mash everything together with a fork.

- Spread the avocado mash over the toast. Arrange the smoked trout or goat's cheese over the top of the avocado. Scatter a few extra dill leaves over the top and sprinkle with some more smoked paprika, then serve.

Roast Squash Wedges

An irresistible – and quick – way of roasting squash and the wedges keep well in the fridge for up to 5 days. My children are particularly fond of these.

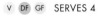 SERVES 4   176 calories

1kg squash, such as coquina, acrorn or butternut
1 tbsp olive oil
Good pinch cayenne pepper
3–4 sprigs fresh thyme, leaves picked
A few sprigs of parsley, to garnish
Sea salt and freshly ground black pepper

For the tahini sauce:
2 tbsp tahini
Zest and juice of ½ lemon

- Preheat the oven to 200°C/400°F/Gas mark 6.

- Slice the squash in half or cut into quarters where the neck meets the bulbous part. Slice the stalk end off the top of the neck (if it's still on it), then slice the neck in half and cut each half into semicircles or wedges around 1.5cm thick.

- Cut the bulbous end in half, and scoop out and discard the seeds. Cut this section in half again, then cut into wedges, around the same size as the others.

- Rub all the pieces with the oil then lay them in a roasting tin, making sure they are in an even layer, and sprinkle over the cayenne pepper. Scatter the thyme leaves over the top, then season well. Roast in the oven for 30 minutes, until tender and until a fork can be easily pushed into the flesh.

- Put the tahini in a bowl and stir in the lemon zest and juice. Add 2–3 tablespoons of water to thin it down – it will transform from a paste into a milky sauce.

- When the squash is ready, transfer it to a large serving bowl. Drizzle with the tahini sauce, scatter over the parsley and serve.

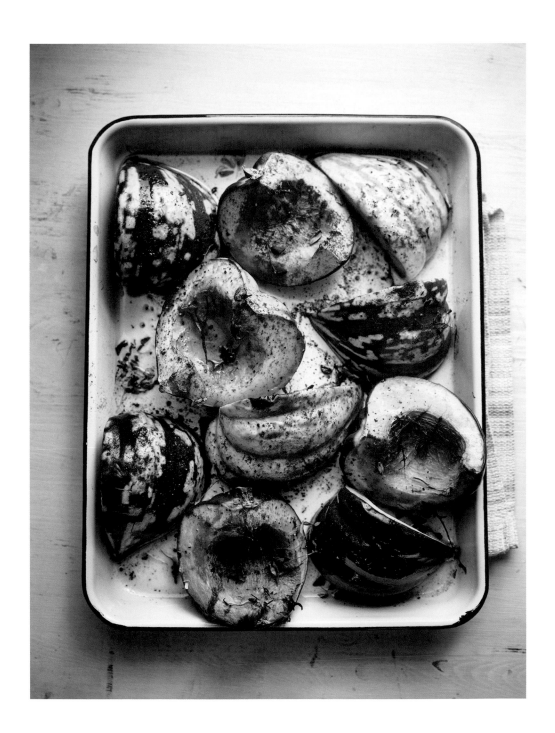

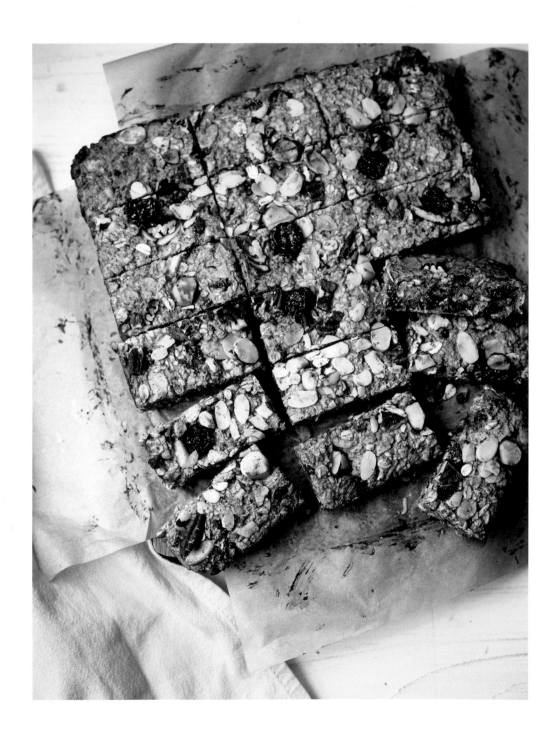

Tropical Energy Bars

These baked flapjack-style bars contain very little honey but some natural sweetness comes from the dried fruit. They're a nourishing afternoon pick-me-up, and because they're so dense you won't be reaching out for more. Wrapped tightly in cling film, they freeze well and you can take out a bar when you need it. It will thaw at room temperature in about an hour.

V   MAKES 18   200 calories per bar

For the dry mix:
A little oil or butter, for greasing
150g jumbo oats
50g buckwheat oats
50g barley flakes
50g flaked almonds
50g brazil nuts, roughly chopped
50g pecan nuts, roughly chopped
100g dried figs, chopped
50g dried cherries
2 tsp mixed spice
Good pinch sea salt

For the wet mix:
200g peeled ripe bananas
50g raw organic honey
50g Smooth Almond and Cinnamon Butter
   (see page 121)
3 eggs
50g unsalted butter, melted and cooled

- Preheat the oven to 200°C/400°F/Gas mark 6. Lightly oil or butter a 20cm square tin and line with baking parchment.

- Put half the jumbo oats, the buckwheat oats and the barley flakes into a food processor and pulse a couple of times, until the mixture has broken down and the flakes are slightly more finely ground.

- Tip the mixture into a bowl, then add the remaining dry ingredients and stir everything together. Put the bananas, honey and almond butter into the food processor and whizz until the mixture turns into a purée. Add the eggs and whizz again to combine.

- Tip the wet mix into the bowl of dry ingredients, add the cooled melted butter and mix everything together really well.

- Spoon into the prepared tin and level the top. Bake for 20–25 minutes, until golden on the top and a skewer inserted into the centre comes out clean. Lift the flapjack square out of the tin on to a cooling rack, and allow to cool completely. Transfer to a board and cut into 18 small bars.

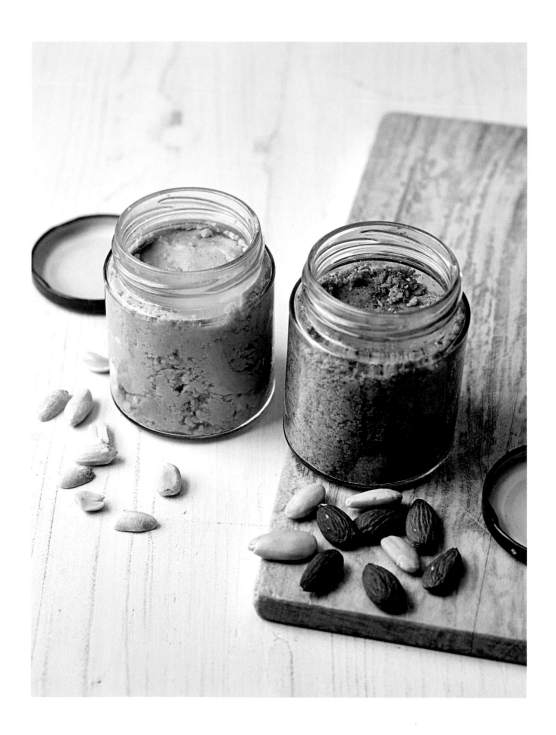

Nut Butters

All my family love nut butters and I've discovered that they're really easy to make at home. I'm a big fan of almond butter, as it's a high-protein skin treat, packed with vitamin E, but my children's favourite is the peanut butter. To sterilise jars, wash them well, then put them in the sink. Pour boiling water into them and the lids. Leave the jars for a few minutes, then carefully tip the water out. The jars dry instantly as the water is so hot and are ready to go. Fill immediately with the nut butter.

Chunky Peanut Butter

V DF GF MAKES 300G   87 calories (per 15g)

300g unsalted peanuts
½ tsp sea salt

- Put the peanuts in a large frying pan and toast over a gentle heat for about 5 minutes, until golden. Keep tossing the pan every now and then to ensure that they're all evenly coloured. Once toasted, allow the nuts to cool a little.

- Transfer half the nuts to a food processor and whizz half until roughly chopped. Tip into a bowl. Add the remaining nuts to the food processor with the salt and whizz until smooth and butter-like.

- Put the chopped nuts back in, and whizz very briefly to combine. Spoon into a sterilised jar, and seal. Store in the fridge for up to 2 weeks.

LIZ'S TIP

For a raw nut butter, don't toast the nuts first, just go straight to the second step to prepare the nuts.

Smooth Almond and Cinnamon Butter

V DF GF MAKES 300G   95 calories (per 15g)

150g whole almonds (with skins)
150g blanched almonds
2 tsp ground cinnamon
Good pinch sea salt

- Put all the almonds in a frying pan and toast for a few minutes, until golden. Make sure they don't burn.

- Cool the almonds a little, then transfer to a food processor and add the cinnamon and salt. Pulse first to break down the nuts, then continue to whizz the mixture until smooth. Depending on how sharp the blades of your food processor are, this takes around 30 minutes of whizzing, scraping down the sides and whizzing again until the nuts are fully ground down, so be patient.

- Spoon into a sterilised jar and cover with a lid. Enjoy within 2 weeks.

White Bean Hummus with a Tahini Swirl and Two Toppings

Make one or both of these toppings to garnish your hummus as you like. I also like to serve the hummus in a wide dish and put the pomegranate topping on one half and the kale topping on the other. As you eat you can scoop up a bit of each!

V DF GF SERVES 4   250 calories

400g can white beans, such as cannellini, drained

2 tbsp extra virgin olive oil

2 tbsp cold water

Zest and juice of ½ lemon

½ tsp ground coriander (optional)

Sea salt and freshly ground black pepper

For the walnut and pomegranate topping:

15g walnuts, chopped (finely or roughly)

1 tbsp tahini

Seeds from ¼ of a pomegranate

Extra virgin olive oil, for drizzling

For the crispy kale topping:

50g kale

1 tsp olive oil

1–2 tsp freshly grated ginger or good pinch
  ground ginger

2 tsp tahini

Extra virgin olive oil, for drizzling

- Put the white beans, extra virgin olive oil, water, lemon zest and juice and ground coriander, if using, into a food processor. Whizz until really smooth.

- Season the mixture well, whizz again, then taste to check the seasoning. This is the sort of dip that needs to sit for a little while for all the flavours to meld together, so use a spatula to divide it between two bowls, then set aside while you make the toppings.

- For the walnut and pomegranate topping, toast the chopped walnuts in a pan over a medium heat for 2–3 minutes, until they turn golden. Drizzle the tahini over one bowl of hummus, then top with the walnuts, the pomegranate seeds and a little extra oil and seasoning.

- For the crispy kale topping, preheat the grill. Put the kale on a baking sheet and drizzle the oil all over. Massage it into the leaves. Scatter the grated ginger over the top or sprinkle with the ground ginger (or do half and half, as I sometimes do). Grill for 5–8 minutes, until golden. Watch it carefully to make sure it doesn't burn. The leaves that are sprinkled with ground ginger will take less time to crisp up than the others.

- Drizzle the tahini over the other bowl of hummus, then spoon the kale on top and drizzle with a little extra oil and seasoning.

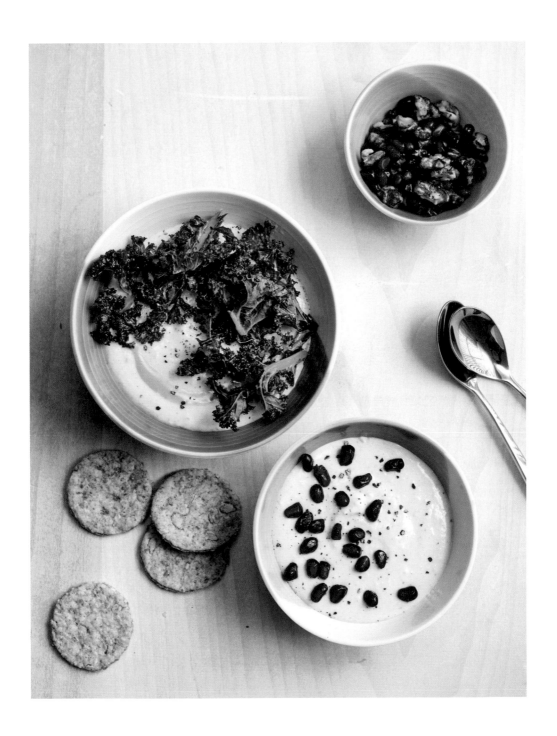

Spelt Crackers

These bite-size crackers have a gorgeously nutty flavour and are made with skin-friendly ingredients such as seeds and olive oil. If you're using sea salt with large crystals it's important to grind it down until fine so it disperses through the mixture.

V DF **MAKES ABOUT 22 CRACKERS**   36 calories per cracker

1 tbsp olive oil, plus extra for brushing

60g jumbo oats

60g spelt flour, plus extra for dusting

½ tsp baking powder

1 tbsp sunflower seeds

1 tsp flaxseeds

Good pinch sea salt

- Preheat the oven to 200°C/400°F/Gas mark 6. Brush a large baking sheet with a little oil.

- Put the jumbo oats into a food processor and pulse once or twice to roughly chop them. Put them in a bowl, then add the spelt flour and baking powder. Add the seeds and the salt, and stir everything together.

- Make a well in the middle, and pour in the olive oil. Add 3–4 tablespoons of cold water and stir again until the mixture starts to form big crumbs.

- Bring the mixture together with your hands and knead lightly to make a ball, then roll out on a lightly floured board until the dough is around 3mm thick. You can do this in two batches if you prefer, by cutting the dough in half first.

- Use a 5cm round cutter to stamp out 16–18 rounds from the dough (or 8–9 rounds if you're just making half). Put the offcuts together and squash the seams to form a flat piece of dough again, then continue to cut out the remaining rounds to make around 22 in total (or around 11).

- Place the rounds on the baking sheet and bake for around 15 minutes, until golden. Transfer to a wire rack to cool, then store in an airtight container for up to 5 days.

Beetroot, Carrot and Apple Crackers

You can make these with the pulp left from making the juice recipe on page 246. They taste great just as they are but are also delicious topped with a little hummus and a few sprigs of watercress. I like to make a big batch of the mixture, then freeze half to bake another time.

V GF   MAKES TWO BATCHES OF 12–15 CRACKERS, PLUS OFFCUTS   29–33 calories per cracker

30g cashews
20g whole almonds
25g flaked almonds
10g linseeds or flaxseeds
1 tsp sea salt
Good grind black pepper

2 good pinches smoked paprika
175g beetroot, apple and carrot pulp (see juice recipe on page 246)
1 tbsp flaxseed oil
1 tbsp water

- Preheat the oven to 180°C/350°F/Gas mark 4. Put the nuts and seeds into a food processor and whizz until the mixture is finely chopped. Add the salt and pepper and smoked paprika and whizz again until the mixture is finely ground.

- Spoon the vegetable pulp into the food processor and add the flaxseed oil and water. Whizz again to combine, then spoon half the mixture on to a large piece of baking parchment. Wrap the remaining half in baking parchment, then in cling film, and freeze for up to 1 month.

- Cover the pulp on the baking parchment with another piece of parchment and roll the mixture out until it's about 3mm thick and measures around 22 x 20cm.

- Peel off the top layer of parchment, and slide the parchment with the rolled-out pulp on it on to a baking sheet. Bake for 15 minutes. Mark into 12–15 squares, each measuring around 5 x 4cm (there may be a few offcuts to nibble on, too). Continue to bake for 15 minutes more until the squares look dry and cooked through – they'll crisp up as they cool. Store in an airtight container for up to 3 days.

LIZ'S TIP

To cook the frozen batch of cracker dough, thaw overnight in a cool room. Roll out between two clean sheets of baking parchment, as in the third step, and complete the recipe.

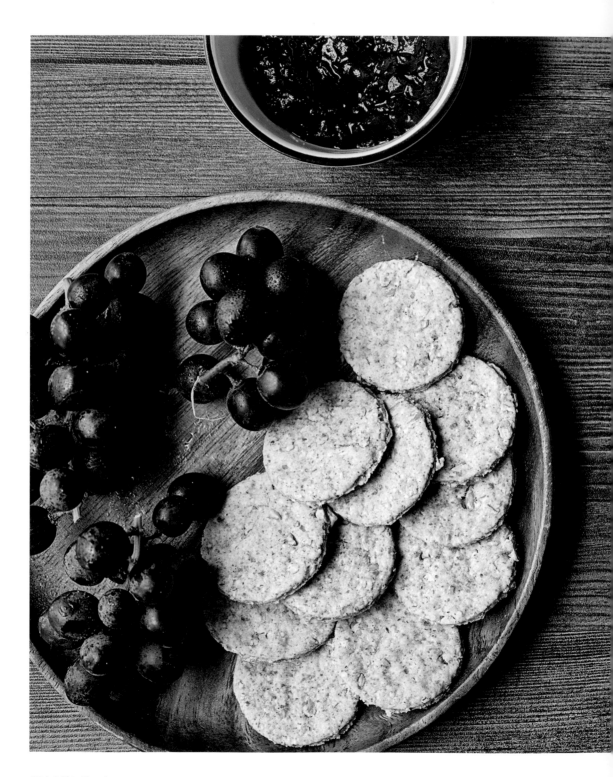

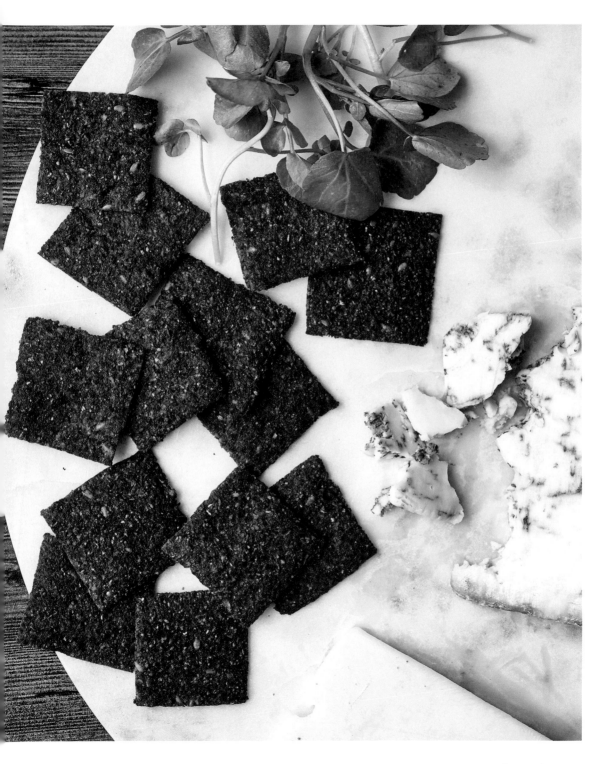

Quail Eggs with Crunchy Sesame Dip

This spicy dip has quite a kick and is the perfect accompaniment to quail eggs or to sliced hard-boiled eggs. I love the spice turmeric, which is traditionally used to help clear and strengthen the skin.

V DF GF   SERVES 4   173 calories

12 quail eggs

1 head chicory or endive (pale yellow/green type)

For the dip:

1 shallot, very finely chopped

2 tsp olive oil or rapeseed oil

2 tsp cider vinegar

1½ tsp sesame seeds

1½ tsp poppy seeds

1½ tsp linseeds

¼ tsp turmeric

Good pinch mild chilli powder

Good pinch garam masala

Sea salt and freshly ground black pepper

- Put the shallot in a small bowl and add the oil and vinegar. Stir together and set aside.

- Lower the quail eggs into a pan of gently boiling water and cook for 2½ minutes. Drain well and cover with cold water. Peel each one, dipping them back into the water again to rinse off any bits of shell.

- Put the seeds and spices in a dry frying pan and heat gently for 1–2 minutes. Stir into the shallot mixture and season well.

- Separate the head of chicory, arrange on a plate with the eggs and serve with the dip.

Crudités with Mustard and Cheese Dip

Crudités make a great snack and when served with this dip they are a perfect dinner party starter, too. The dip is also good on a spelt cracker (see page 124).

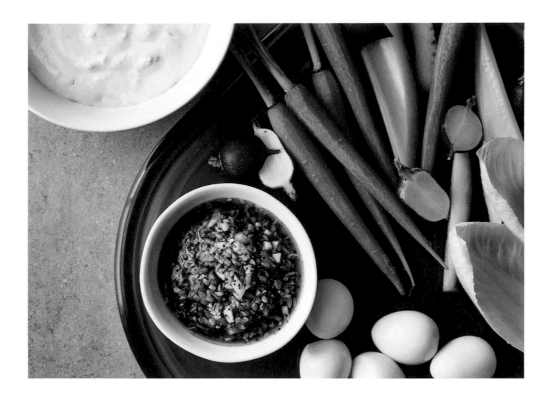

For the mustard and cheese dip:
100g feta, roughly chopped
2 tbsp natural yoghurt
1–2 tbsp whole milk
1–1½ tsp Dijon mustard
2 stoned queen green olives, finely chopped
2 tbsp chopped fresh dill
1 tsp nonpareille capers
4 whole walnuts, finely chopped

¼ tsp white wine vinegar
1 tsp rapeseed oil
Sea salt and freshly ground black pepper

For the crudités:
2 celery sticks, chopped into finger-length batons
5 spring carrots, peeled
¼ cucumber, chopped into finger-length batons
6 radishes, halved

- Put the feta, yoghurt, milk and mustard into a mini food processor and whizz to make a smooth mixture. Season with a pinch of salt and whizz again, adding 1–2 tablespoons of cold water if the mixture is very thick. Spoon into a bowl and set aside.

- Put the olives, dill, capers, walnuts, vinegar and oil into a small bowl and mix everything together, seasoning well. Spoon on top of the dip or fold it in and garnish with an extra grind of pepper.

- Serve the crudités with the dip.

Snack Ideas

These are some of my tried and tested skin-friendly snacks. They're all great for staving off hunger pangs or keeping the hungry hordes going until the next meal!

Blueberry Mess

Put a large handful of blueberries into a bowl and squish with the back of a fork to release the juices. Dust with a pinch of cinnamon. Add 2 heaped tablespoons of Greek yoghurt, then sprinkle with 1 tablespoon of toasted flaked almonds and roughly fold together.

Peach and Dukkah

A twist on the Egyptian dipping condiment, to serve with ripe peaches or nectarines. Finely chop 8 whole hazelnuts. Put them in a small ramekin with a pinch each of cinnamon, ground ginger and freshly grated nutmeg. Stir together. Slice a ripe peach or nectarine into thin wedges and dip into the mix.

Yoghurt, Berry Compote and Nut Butter

So simple, but very filling. Put 2 heaped tablespoons of Greek yoghurt into a small pot. Top with a teaspoonful each of Low-Sugar Berry Compote and Smooth Almond and Cinnamon Butter (see pages 231 and 121 for recipes).

Sweet and Savoury Spelt Cracker Snacks

For the sweet one: spread three Spelt Crackers (see page 124) with a little ricotta or low-fat cream cheese. Top with a small spoonful of Low-Sugar Berry Compote (see page 231) and spread over the cheese to mix.

For the savoury one: take three Spelt Crackers and spread each with a little mashed avocado (around ¼ avocado will be plenty). Top each with halved cherry tomatoes, a pinch of sea salt and a dusting of paprika.

Cucumber and White Bean Hummus

Take a 5cm piece of cucumber, slice it in half lengthways, then scoop out the seeds with a teaspoon. Spoon some White Bean Hummus (see page 122) or ready-made hummus into each channel. Season with a little freshly ground black pepper, then scatter over a few capers and chopped fresh parsley.

Apple and Nut Butter

An oldie, but a goodie! Core then slice an apple into eight pieces. Spread four of them with a little nut butter – peanut is particularly good – then sprinkle with a little cinnamon. Sandwich each together with an unadorned apple slice.

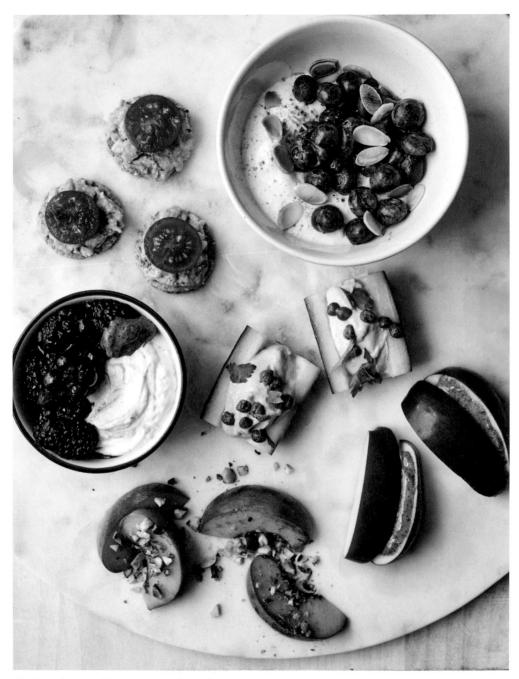

Clockwise from top left: Savoury Spelt Crackers,
Blueberry Mess, Cucumber and White Bean
Hummus, Apple and Nut Butter, Peach and Dukkah,
Yoghurt, Berry Compote and Nut Butter

Liz's Beauty Bombs

Beauty bombs are my way of blasting the skin with a mouthful of tasty, nutritious treats. Sweet and savoury, each one is packed with nutrients that make our skin glow. They keep well – either in an airtight container for up to 5 days or in the freezer for up to 1 month. To thaw, just take one out and put it on a plate, and it'll be ready to eat in 15–30 minutes.

Berry and Seed Beauty Bombs

V DF MAKES 8–10   64–80 calories

15g pumpkin seeds
15g sunflower seeds
10g sesame seeds
30g unsweetened
   dried sour cherries
30g unsweetened
   dried cranberries

20g barley flakes
25g sultanas
50g dates, stoned
Pinch sea salt
Squeeze orange juice

- Put the pumpkin seeds, sunflower seeds and sesame seeds into a frying pan and place over a medium heat. Cook for 3–4 minutes until the sesame seeds start to pop and the sunflower and pumpkin seeds turn golden.

- Tip the seeds into a food processor and add the sour cherries, cranberries, barley flakes, sultanas, dates and sea salt. Whizz to combine the ingredients together, scraping the mixture down halfway through. Add the orange juice and whizz again until the mixture starts to come together.

- Tip the combined mixture into a bowl or on to a board and divide it into eight to ten evenly sized pieces. Roll each piece into a ball, then transfer to a small airtight container to store.

Tropical Beauty Bombs

V DF GF MAKES 8–10   71–90 calories

75g dried apricots,
   roughly chopped
25g unsweetened
   dried mango,
   roughly chopped

25g ground almonds
25g coconut flakes
25g whole almonds
½ cm slice fresh root
   ginger, peeled and
   grated

- Put the dried apricots, dried mango, ground almonds, coconut flakes, whole almonds and ginger into a food processor.

- Turn the food processor on to high to blend all the ingredients together. Stop it every now and then and push the mixture down with a spatula to make sure everything is evenly combined.

- Tip the combined mixture into a bowl or on to a board and divide it into eight to ten evenly sized pieces. Roll each piece into a ball, then transfer to a small airtight container to store.

Date and Dark Chocolate Beauty Bombs

V DF MAKES 8–10   75–93 calories

100g ready-to-eat dried dates
30g jumbo oats
20g dark chocolate (over 80% cocoa solids, or cocoa nibs – see tip)
30g walnut halves
½ tsp ground cinnamon
1 tsp linseeds
2 tsp cold water

- Put the dates, oats, chocolate and walnut halves into a food processor. (If you're using cocoa nibs, leave them out of the processor at this stage.)

- Add the cinnamon, linseeds and water. Turn the processor on to high and whizz the mixture until smooth. Scrape the mixture down halfway through so that all the ingredients are chopped up evenly.

- Tip the combined mixture into a bowl or on to a board and divide it into eight to ten evenly sized pieces. Roll each piece into a ball, then transfer to a small airtight container to store.

LIZ'S TIP

If you're using cocoa nibs, put the mixture into a bowl and then add the cocoa nibs. Work the nibs evenly into the mixture by squeezing and kneading everything together, then complete the recipe.

Over page: Beauty Bombs clockwise from top left: Berry and Seed, Tropical, Date and Dark Chocolate and Savoury

Savoury Beauty Bombs

V DF MAKES 10   90 calories

50g chickpeas, drained
50g walnuts
50g jumbo or rolled oats
50g peeled and grated carrot
10g parsley
Good pinch chilli flakes (optional)
1 egg
2 tbsp sesame seeds
Sea salt and freshly ground black pepper

- Preheat the oven to 200°C/400°F/Gas mark 6.

- Put the chickpeas, walnuts, oats, carrot and parsley in a food processor and whizz to blend everything together. Season well and add the chilli flakes. Whizz again to combine, then taste to adjust the seasoning.

- Add the egg and blend again to mix the egg into the other ingredients. Spoon the mixture into a bowl and divide into ten equal portions, each around 25g, and roll them into balls. Spread the sesame seeds on a plate and roll each ball in them.

- Space the balls well apart on a baking tray and bake for 15 minutes. Allow to cool, then enjoy. They'll keep for up to 3 days in an airtight container in the fridge, or wrap in cling film, store in an airtight container and freeze for up to 2 weeks.

LIZ'S TIP

Try adding chopped feta or hard goat's cheese. You only need 40g to give a good flavour. Either break the cheese up and combine it with the mixture then roll it into 30g balls, or, if you're using a hard cheese, grate it and mix it in. Roll in sesame seeds and bake as above.

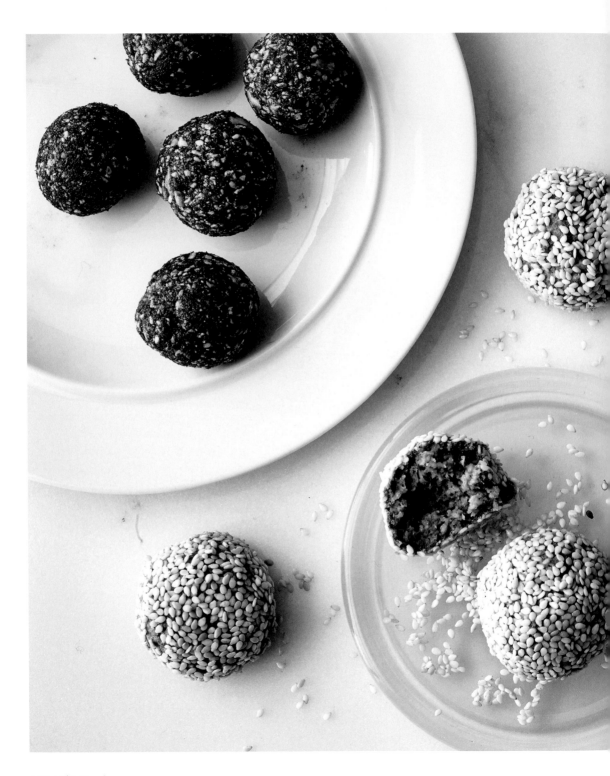

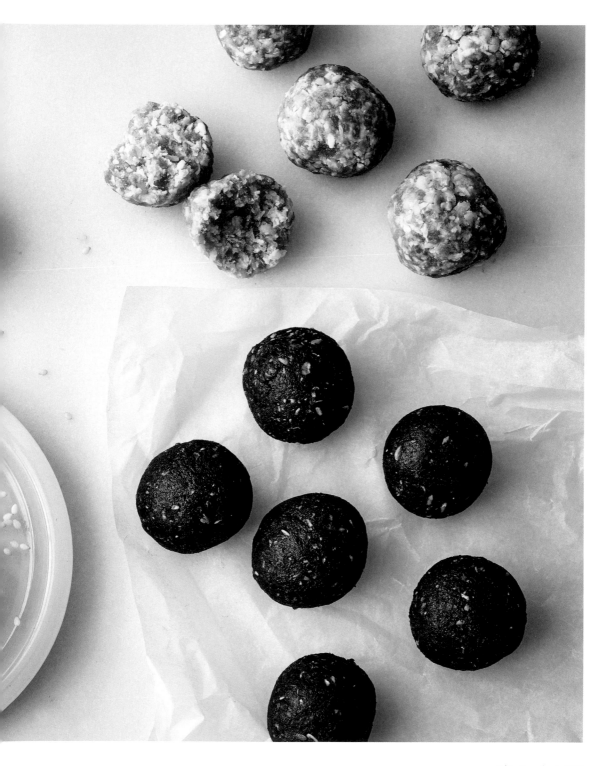

LIGHT MEALS

White Bean, Watercress, Fennel and Tuna Salad

Fast food can be healthy! I often make this salad with a jar of tuna and canned beans for a quick lunch but I also love it with fresh tuna for a special feast with family and friends.

 DF GF SERVES 4   260 calories

150g green beans
300g yellowfin tuna steak (or use the equivalent
    weight of tuna from a jar, drained of any oil)
1 tsp olive or rapeseed oil
100g watercress
1 small fennel bulb, with fronds
½ cucumber
400g can white beans, such as cannellini or
    haricot, drained

For the dressing:
Zest and juice of ½ lemon
3 tbsp extra virgin olive oil
1 tsp Dijon mustard
2 tsp nonpareille capers
Sea salt and freshly ground black pepper

- Make the dressing by whisking all the ingredients together in a large salad bowl with 1 teaspoon of water and a little salt and pepper.

- Put the green beans in a saucepan, and cover with water. Bring to the boil and cook for 2–3 minutes until just tender. Drain well and put the beans into the bowl with the dressing.

- Season the tuna well. Heat the oil in a frying pan and fry the tuna steak for 3 minutes on each side. This will leave the tuna pink in the middle. If you prefer it well cooked, continue to cook for another minute on each side. Put the tuna on a board and slice thinly.

- Roughly chop the watercress and add it to the salad bowl. Use a mandolin or sharp knife to finely slice the fennel bulb and add that, too. Half the cucumber lengthways, and run a spoon down the centre to remove the seeds. Slice into half-moons and add them to the bowl.

- Add the beans and toss everything together, then arrange the tuna on top and serve.

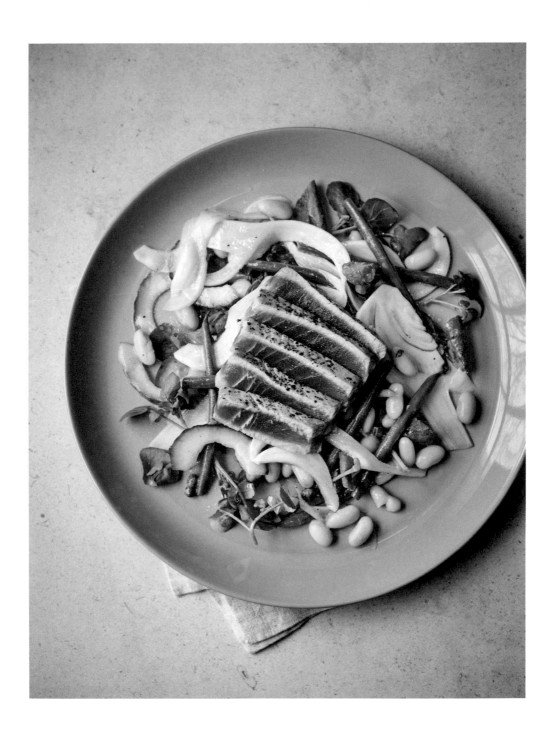

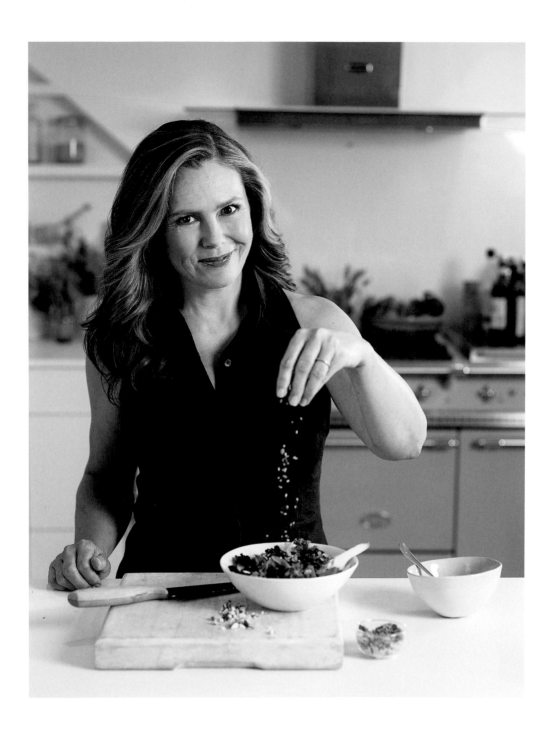

Kale, Beetroot and Fennel Slaw with a Spiced Dressing

Here's my modern take on coleslaw, featuring three of my favourite vegetables – kale, beetroot and fennel (which are anti-inflammatory, iron-rich and vitamin C-rich respectively). I've chopped the kale finely so it seasons the salad like a herb, and teamed it with wafer-thin fennel and matchsticks of beetroot for crunch. This slaw is perfect on its own for lunch or can also be served alongside grilled mackerel, an oily fish packed with Omega-3, the all-important fatty acid essential for good skin.

V 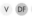 GF   SERVES 2   280 calories

1 small fennel bulb
1 beetroot
25g kale
Small handful mint
20g whole almonds, chopped
1 tbsp mixed seeds: pumpkin, sunflower, sesame
    and linseeds

For the dressing:
½ tsp fennel seeds
½ tsp mustard seeds
½ tsp coriander seeds
2 tbsp extra virgin olive oil
Juice of ½ lemon
Good pinch freshly ground black pepper

- Use a mandolin or a very sharp knife to slice the fennel very thinly into a bowl.

- Peel the beetroot and chop it into matchsticks. Spoon the beetroot on top of the fennel.

- Chop the kale finely – as if you were chopping a herb – and do the same with the mint, keeping a few of the smaller mint leaves whole, and sprinkle over the bowl. Scatter the almonds and mixed seeds over the top.

- Heat the fennel, mustard and coriander seeds in a frying pan for 2 minutes, until the mustard seeds start to pop. Spoon into a pestle and mortar, add the pepper and lightly crush. Put the crushed seeds and pepper into a bowl with the olive oil and lemon juice, and whisk together.

- Spoon the dressing over the salad, then toss everything together and serve.

The New Chicken Liver Salad

Chicken livers are nourishing, cheap and delicious. I love them in this salad with its tangy mustardy dressing.

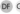 DF GF SERVES 4   242 calories

8 mini plum tomatoes, halved
1 tbsp olive oil, plus extra for brushing
150g green beans, halved
1 small red onion, sliced
350g chicken livers
Pinch chilli flakes
1 tsp good-quality balsamic vinegar
2 little gem lettuces
1 tbsp chopped fresh parsley

30g rocket
Salt and freshly ground black pepper

For the grainy mustard dressing:
3 tbsp extra virgin olive oil
1 tsp grainy mustard
1 tbsp chopped fresh chives
1 tbsp white wine vinegar

- Preheat the grill. Lay the tomatoes on a baking sheet, brush them with oil and season well. Grill for 5–10 minutes, until roasted and starting to shrivel.

- Bring a small saucepan of water to the boil and cook the green beans until tender. Drain well.

- Mix all the ingredients together for the dressing, and set aside.

- Put 1 tablespoon of olive oil in a large frying pan and add the sliced onion. Cook for 5 minutes until it is starting to soften, then add the chicken livers to the pan and cook for a further 5 minutes, until the livers are completely cooked through. Sprinkle over the chilli flakes and drizzle over the balsamic vinegar.

- Separate the lettuce leaves and arrange them on a large platter or in a salad bowl. Scatter over the parsley, rocket, green beans and tomatoes, then spoon over the liver and onion mixture. Drizzle over the dressing, and serve.

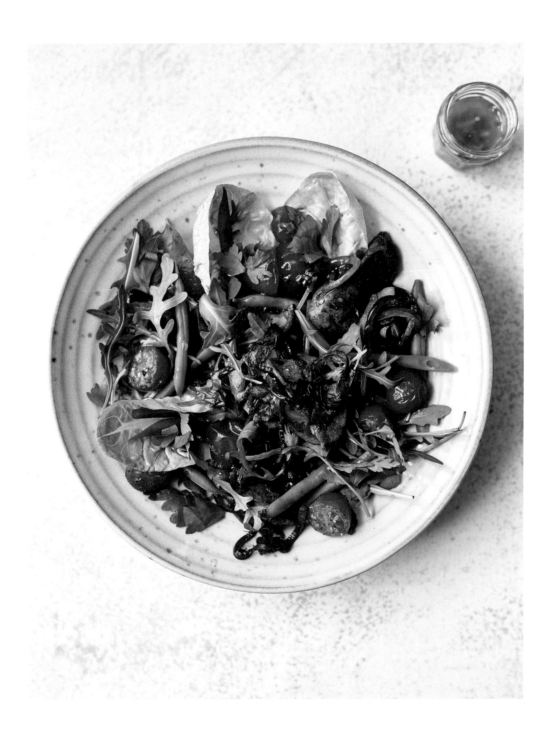

Broccoli and Feta Crustless Quiche

I do love a quiche but don't like to eat too much pastry so this recipe is perfect – all the flavour and fun without the stodge. Broccoli is a great skin-friendly vegetable, rich in vitamin C and folic acid as well as minerals such as calcium, iron and potassium.

V GF   SERVES 4–6   176 calories

350g broccoli, stalks separated
2 spring onions, finely chopped
8 medium eggs
100g feta, chopped

2 tbsp chopped fresh parsley
4 cherry tomatoes, halved
Salt and freshly ground black pepper

- Preheat the oven to 200°C/400°F/Gas mark 6.

- Bring a large saucepan of water to the boil, and add the broccoli. Cook for 3–5 minutes, until the broccoli is tender. Add the spring onions to the pan and cook for another 30 seconds – this just blanches the spring onions, to take the raw edge off the flavour. Drain well, then arrange the broccoli florets and spring onions in a round 20cm flexible cake tin.

- Beat the eggs in a bowl and add the feta, parsley and seasoning. Whisk again to break the feta into smaller chunks. Spoon the mixture over the broccoli, then arrange the halved cherry tomatoes over the top.

- Bake in the oven for about 35 minutes, until the egg has set and the top is golden. Great served hot or cold.

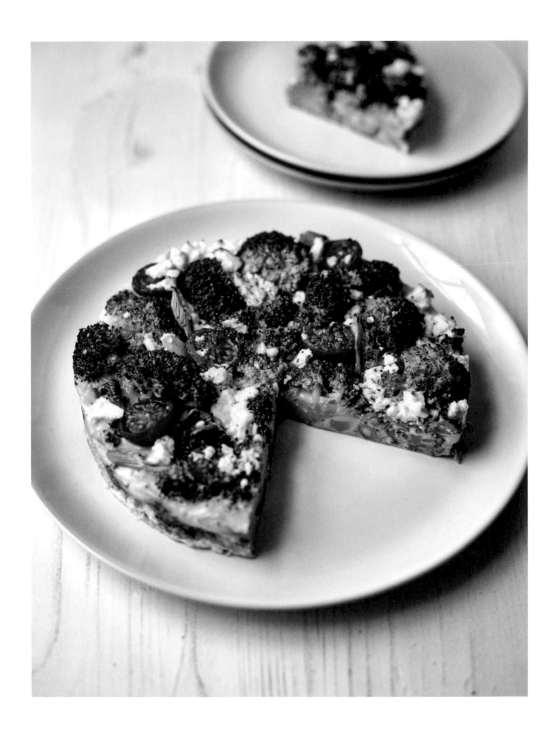

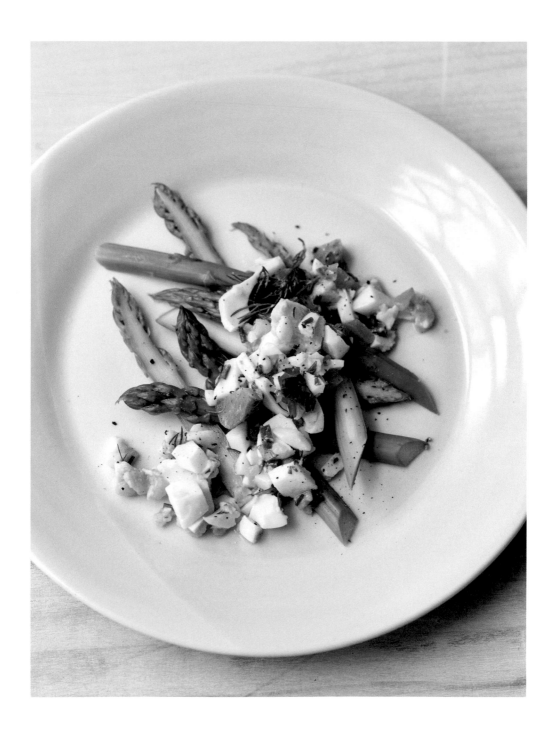

Asparagus with Mimosa

Steamed spears of asparagus are seasoned with this classic dressing made by chopping the whites of hard-boiled eggs and tossing them with capers and gherkins, then grating over the hard-boiled yolks. Serve with freshly chopped herbs – a perfect early summer treat.

V 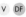 SERVES 4   154 calories

4 eggs
16 asparagus spears
1 tbsp capers
4 gherkins, sliced

1 tbsp each chopped fresh parsley, chives and dill
2 tbsp extra virgin olive oil
1 tsp white wine vinegar
Sea salt and freshly ground black pepper

- Bring a small pan of water to the boil and cook the eggs for 7–8 minutes, until hard-boiled. Put the eggs in a bowl and cover with cold water. Allow them to cool, then crack the shells and peel them.

- Lay the asparagus in a shallow frying pan and cover with a little water. Cover the pan with a lid, and bring it to the boil. Turn the heat down low and cook for 3–5 minutes or until you can push a knife into a stem and it feels tender. Drain well.

- Cut around each peeled egg and carefully remove the white. Finely chop the white, and put it in a bowl with the capers, gherkins and fresh herbs. Add the oil, vinegar and seasoning. Toss together.

- Divide the asparagus between four plates, then spoon the egg white mixture over the top. Grate the yolks over the top, and serve.

Courgette, Carrot and Nut Loaf

This is a light modern version of the trad nut roast. Serve with some salad and green veggies for lunch or supper or pop a slice in your lunch box.

v SERVES 4   360 calories

A little olive oil, for greasing
1 courgette, grated
1 carrot, grated
1 corn on the cob
1 spring onion, finely chopped
60g goat's cheese, chopped
50g almonds, finely chopped

35g Brazil nuts, chopped
2 tbsp chopped fresh parsley
4 sundried tomatoes, finely chopped
75g sourdough or wholemeal bread, chopped
3 eggs
Sea salt and freshly ground black pepper

- Preheat the oven to 200°C/400°F/Gas mark 6. Lightly oil a 900g loaf tin and line it with baking parchment.

- Line a sieve with kitchen paper, put the grated courgette and carrot into it and squeeze out as much moisture as possible. Tip the veg into a bowl. Run a knife all around the corn cob to release the kernels and put them in the bowl too, along with the spring onion, goat's cheese, nuts, parsley, sundried tomatoes and bread.

- Beat the eggs in a separate bowl and season well. Add to the vegetable mixture and fold everything together. Spoon the mixture into the prepared loaf tin and bake for 45 minutes, until the top is golden and the egg has cooked through and set. Cover the loaf tin with foil for the last 15 minutes of cooking if the top looks as if it is browning too much.

- Slice and serve with green beans and salad.

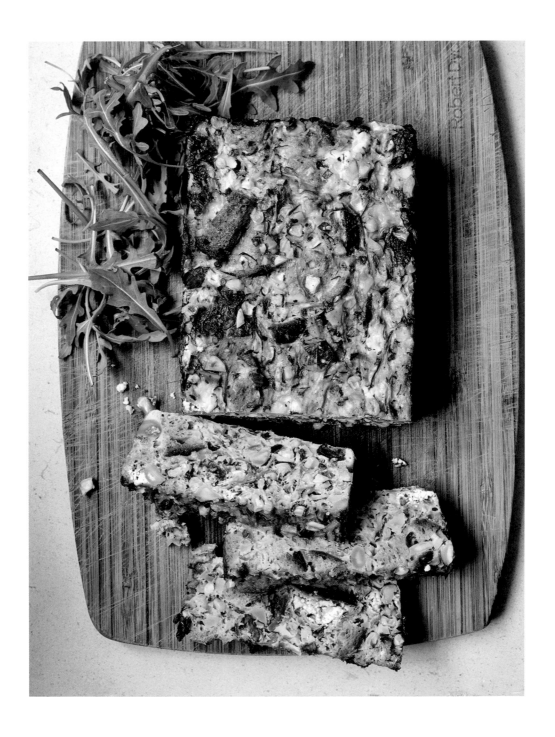

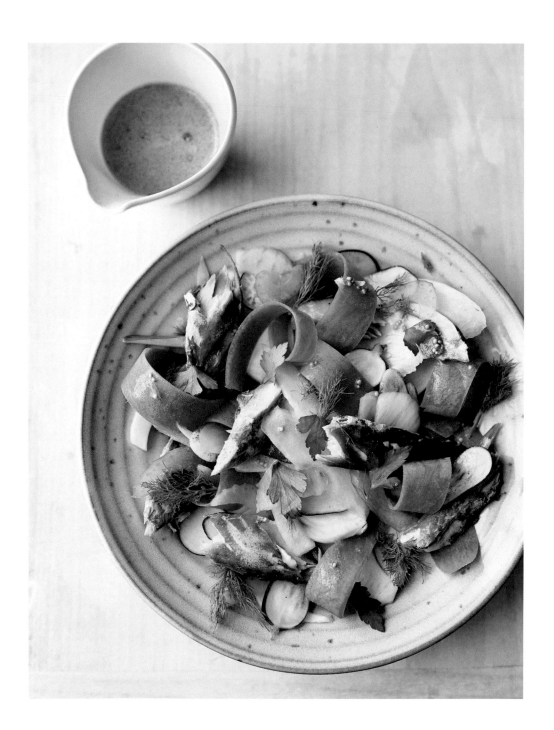

Smoked Mackerel with Poppy Seed Salad

As there are no leaves in this salad to go soggy it can be made in advance if you like. The vegetables are happy marinating in the lemon dressing until you're ready to eat. I could cheerfully eat this every day – it's that good!

 SERVES 4   386 calories

4 fillets good-quality smoked mackerel

For the salad:
1 small fennel bulb
1 large carrot
4 pink radishes
½ daikon or white radish
1 celery stick
1 tbsp chopped fresh parsley

For the lemony dressing:
2 tbsp extra virgin olive oil
Zest and juice of ½ lemon
1 tsp Dijon mustard
2 tsp poppy or mustard seeds
Sea salt and freshly ground black pepper

- Use a mandolin or very sharp knife to finely slice the fennel into a bowl; set aside any fronds. Do the same with the carrot, radishes, daikon and celery. Scatter any fennel fronds over the mixture, with the parsley.

- Whisk together the extra virgin olive oil, lemon zest and juice, Dijon mustard and seeds, and season well.

- Pour the dressing over the salad and serve with the mackerel.

Courgette and Swiss Chard Soup

Generous handfuls of herbs make this veggie soup really fragrant and tasty. It freezes well so you might like to pop some in the freezer for another time.

V   SERVES 8   82 calories

2 tbsp olive oil
25g unsalted butter
100g leek, finely chopped
1 garlic clove, sliced
750g courgettes, finely chopped
350g chard, chopped
Freshly grated nutmeg

1 litre vegetable stock
10g fresh dill, plus extra to serve
10g fresh parsley
Salt and freshly ground black pepper

- Heat the oil and butter gently in a large saucepan, and as soon as the butter has melted, stir in the chopped leek. Add 1 tablespoon of water, then cook over a low heat for 5 minutes.

- Stir in the garlic and courgettes and continue to cook for 10 minutes, stirring every now and then. Add the chard and stir everything together again. Season well with the salt, pepper and nutmeg, and cook for 2–3 minutes until the chard leaves have started to wilt.

- Pour in the stock, cover with a lid and bring to the boil. Simmer for 10–15 minutes, until all the vegetables have cooked through. Stir in the dill and parsley.

- Allow to cool a little, then use a hand-held stick blender to blend half of the soup, leaving a few bits in there for texture. The rest of the soup can be frozen. Serve with extra dill, plus a sprinkling of black pepper.

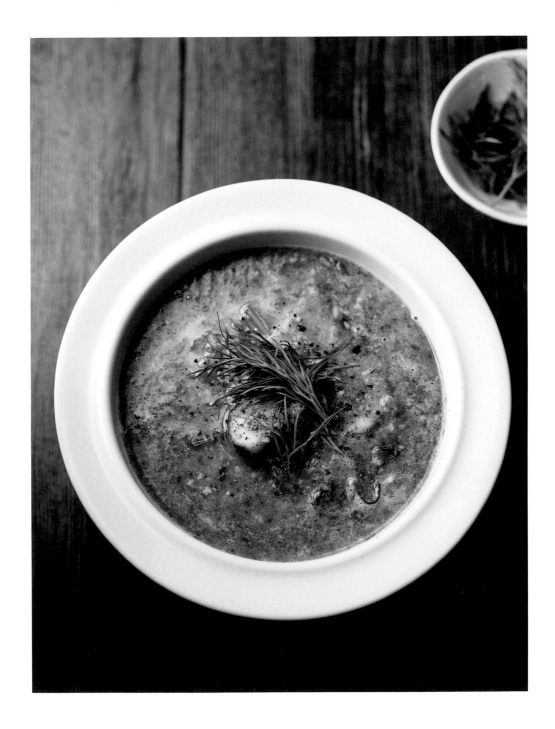

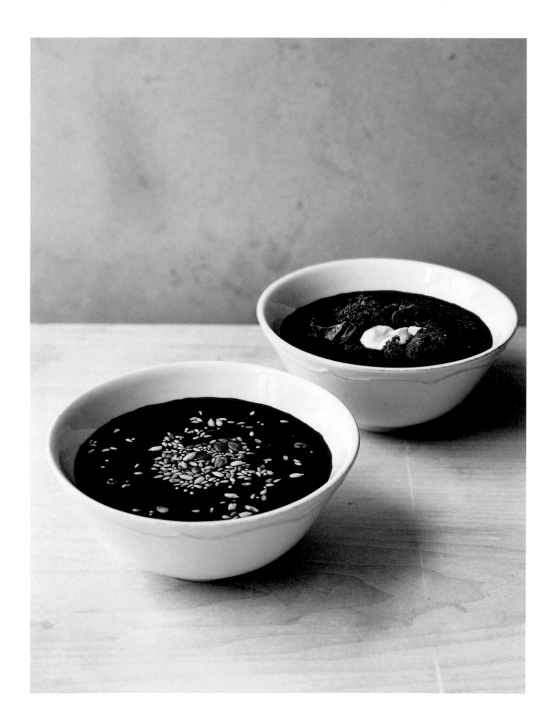

Beetroot Soup with Crispy Kale

Beetroot makes wonderful soup as it not only looks beautiful but is also very nutritious. I love the kale garnish but I've added a crunchy toasted seed recipe as well for when you feel like a change. Beetroot is great for stamina, so eat this on gym days.

v SERVES 8   128 calories

2 tbsp olive oil
1 onion, finely chopped
2 celery sticks, finely chopped
1 large carrot, finely chopped
800g beetroot, roughly chopped
1 garlic clove, sliced
1cm coin fresh root ginger, finely chopped

1.5 litres vegetable stock
Sea salt and freshly ground black pepper

For the crispy kale:
50g kale
1 tsp olive oil
2 tbsp Greek yoghurt

- Heat the oil in a large saucepan and add the onion, celery and carrot. Add 2 tablespoons of water – this is to prevent the vegetables from burning. Cook over a low heat for 10–15 minutes, until the vegetables have softened and caramelised.

- Add the beetroot, garlic and ginger and cook for 1 minute. Pour the stock over the top, season well, cover and simmer for 15 minutes, until the beetroot is tender.

- While the soup is simmering, make the crispy kale garnish. Preheat the grill. Spread the kale out on a board and drizzle with the oil. Season well, then grill until the kale starts to crisp up.

- Allow the beetroot mixture to cool a little, then whizz in a blender or with a hand-held stick blender. Reheat, then serve topped with the kale and a swirl of Greek yoghurt.

An alternative garnish:

- Toast 1 tablespoon of mixed seeds (such as nigella, pumpkin, mustard, sunflower and linseeds) for 1 minute, then divide them between the soup bowls and drizzle with a little olive oil.

Roasted Vegetable Soup

Roasting the vegetables first gives this soup a wonderfully rich flavour, and adding stock to the roasting tin means that the veg stay moist and don't shrivel up.

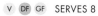 V DF GF **SERVES 8**

100 calories

2 white onions, quartered
3 celery sticks, roughly chopped
2 red peppers, halved and deseeded
1 squash (around 800g–1kg)
2 garlic cloves, unpeeled

2 sprigs rosemary
2 tbsp flaxseed or olive oil
1.2 litres hot vegetable stock
Salt and freshly ground black pepper

- Preheat the oven to 200°C/400°F/Gas mark 6.

- Put the onions, celery and peppers into a roasting tin, so that everything fits quite snugly.

- Slice the squash in half and discard the seeds, then cut it into chunks. There's no need to peel, as it will soften as you roast it and should purée in the blender at the end.

- Add the garlic to the tin with the rosemary, then drizzle over the oil and toss everything together. Pour 400ml of the vegetable stock into the bottom of the tin and roast for 45–50 minutes, or until the vegetables are tender, tossing them halfway through the cooking time.

- Spoon the vegetables into a food processor. Squeeze out the garlic and strip the leaves from the rosemary and add that, too. Add half of the remaining stock, season well and whizz until smooth.

- Return the mixture to a large saucepan with the remaining vegetable stock and bring to the boil, and simmer until you are ready to serve.

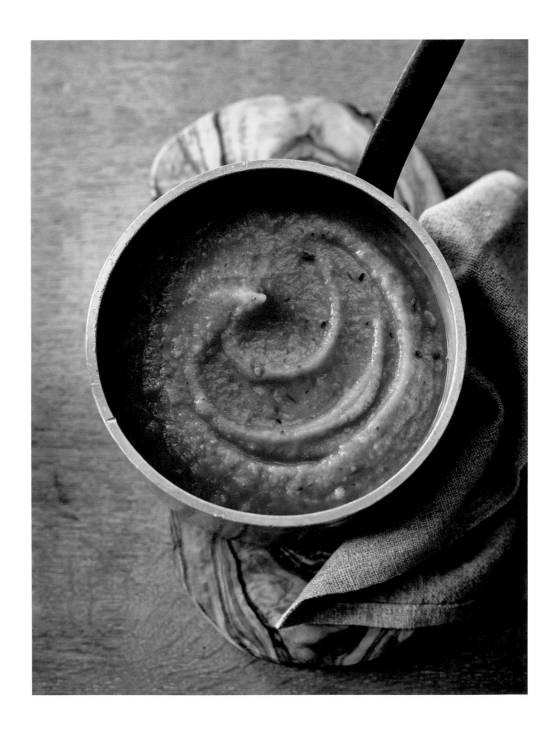

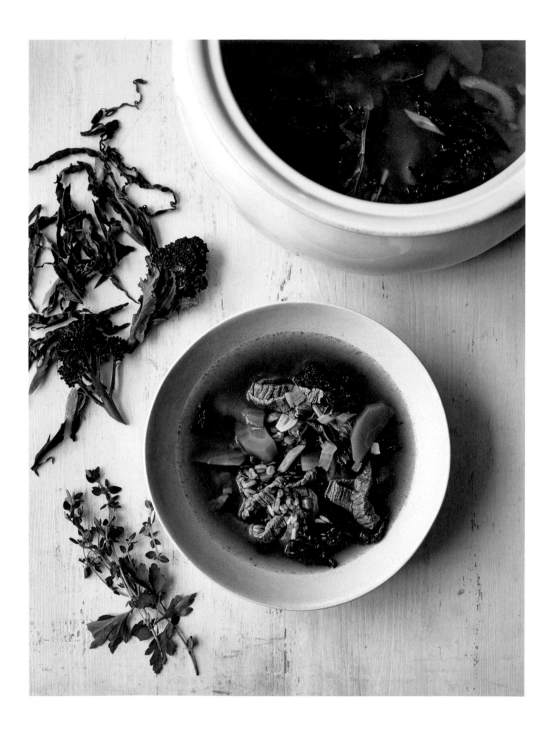

Liz's Beauty Broth

This fabulous soup is a little like Scotch broth but instead of braising the beef in the broth, I add thin strips of minute steak at the end. The steak is first tossed in skin-friendly cayenne pepper to give it a bit of a kick. A really warming dish – great for Sunday supper after a bracing wintery walk!

DF **SERVES 4–6**   231–346 calories

1½ tbsp olive or rapeseed oil
1 onion, finely chopped
2 carrots, finely chopped
2 celery sticks, finely chopped
1 garlic clove, sliced
A few thyme sprigs
50g pearl barley
1.5 litres hot beef stock (made from 6 cubes of
   Beef Stock, see page 239)

50g short-grain brown rice
50g green lentils
6 cavolo nero leaves, chopped
100g sprouting broccoli, chopped
400g minute steak
¼ tsp cayenne pepper (less if preferred)
10g chopped fresh parsley
Sea salt and freshly ground pepper

• Heat the oil in a large saucepan and add the onion, carrots and celery, with 2 tablespoons of cold water. Stir together and sauté for 10 minutes, until the vegetables start to soften and turn golden.Stir in the garlic and thyme and cook for 1 minute, then add the barley, followed by the stock. Season well. Put a lid on the pan and bring to the boil. Simmer for 30 minutes.

• Stir in the rice and lentils and continue to simmer for 20 minutes, then stir in the cavolo nero and broccoli and cook for a further 5 minutes. Fish out the spriggy parts of the thyme – by this stage the leaves will have come away from them and flavoured the soup.

• Cut the minute steak into thin strips, toss with the cayenne pepper and season well. Drop the strips into the soup and nudge them under the surface so they poach in the hot liquor for a minute or so, and cook until the meat is just tender. Stir in the parsley and serve.

LIZ'S TIP

For a slightly cheaper cut, try beef skirt, which you can cook in one of two ways. If you prefer steak-style strips as above, use the same weight but cut into four pieces, following the grain. Brush with cayenne then fry in a little oil, until golden and the outside is sealed, turning as necessary. Slice thinly then drop into the soup before serving. Another way is to braise the beef. After stirring in the garlic and thyme in the second step, brush the beef skirt with the cayenne, then put it into the pan. Pour over the stock and simmer for 30 minutes first, then stir in the barley and continue to cook following the method above.

Buckwheat Noodle Salad

There are plenty of skin-friendly ingredients in this crunchy salad. Seaweed is particularly nutritious, containing iron, iodine, vitamin C and chlorophyll, too. I like Japanese arame, which looks a bit like big tea leaves when it's in the packet, but doubles in volume once soaked.

 SERVES 4   329 calories

200g soba (buckwheat) noodles
5g seaweed
1 red pepper, halved and deseeded
2 spring onions, ends removed
1 carrot
100g mangetout, trimmed
100g green beans, trimmed

For the pumpkin dressing:
2 tbsp extra virgin olive oil
1 tbsp flaxseed oil
1 tsp toasted sesame oil
Juice of 1 lime
1 tsp soy sauce
2 tsp cold water
10g parsley
1 tbsp pumpkin seeds, toasted
15g unsalted peanuts, toasted
Sea salt and freshly ground black pepper

- Soak the noodles and the seaweed according to the packet intructions.

- Prepare the vegetables: finely shred the pepper into thin strips. Do the same with the spring onions. Chop the carrot into matchstick-size shreds. Halve the mangetout lengthways, and do the same with the green beans. Put all the vegetables in a steamer and steam until tender – this will take around 3–5 minutes. You still want there to be a little crunch.

- Put all the ingredients for the dressing in a mini food processor, and season well. Whizz until smooth.

- Drain the buckwheat noodles and the seaweed, and mix together. Divide between four bowls, and do the same with the vegetables. Drizzle over the dressing, and serve.

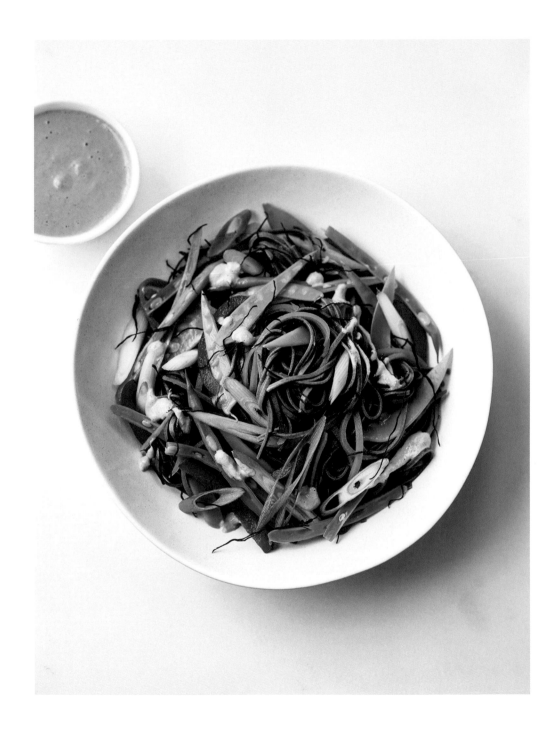

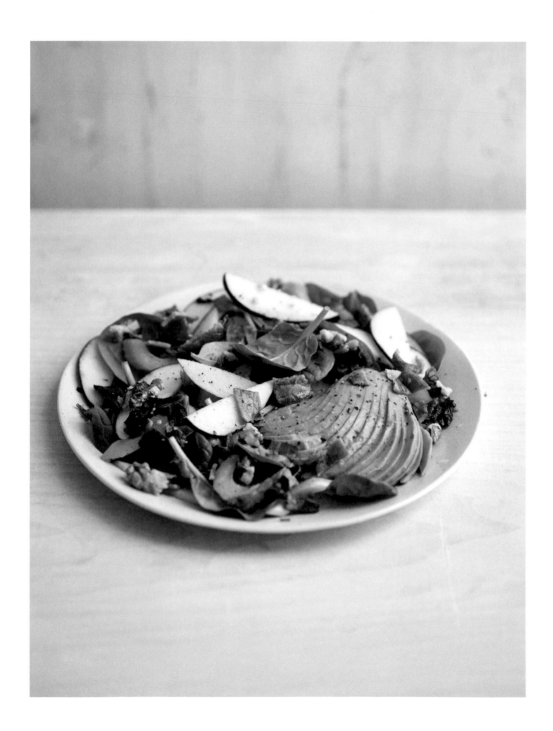

The New Avocado and Bacon Salad

This updated version of a classic combination is lovely on its own or with some cold roast chicken for a quick lunch or supper. A nutty-flavoured English apple, such as Egremont Russet, goes well with the other ingredients in this salad.

DF GF SERVES 4   322 calories

175g back bacon
1 avocado
¼ lemon
2 celery sticks, finely sliced

150g baby leaf spinach, washed well
2 apples
25g walnuts, toasted and roughly chopped
3 tbsp Apple Cider Vinaigrette (see page 237)

- Preheat the grill and cook the bacon until golden. Snip into small pieces.

- Cut the avocado in half, remove the stone and slice the flesh. Squeeze over the lemon to stop it discolouring. Put the avocado slices in a large bowl with the celery and the spinach.

- Core and finely slice the apples, and put them on top, along with the walnuts. Drizzle over the dressing. Scatter the bacon on top and toss everything together.

Baked Beetroot

A favourite of mine, baked beetroot are so easy to cook and I love them with our Sunday roast lamb or with some lamb chops. Beetroot contains many nutrients, including folic acid, magnesium and iron.

V GF SERVES 4   218 calories

4 medium beetroots (around 750g in total), washed

4 shallots, peeled

2 tbsp olive or flaxseed oil

100g feta or crumbly goat's milk cheese, finely chopped

2 sprigs dill, finely chopped, plus extra to serve

1 tbsp pumpkin seeds, toasted

Salt and freshly ground black pepper

- Preheat the oven to 200°C/400°F/Gas mark 6.

- Put the beetroots and shallots into a large piece of foil and drizzle over the oil. Add the dill and season well. Wrap the foil up, put it in a roasting tin and roast for 45 minutes, until the beetroots are tender.

- When the beetroots are ready, cut each bulb into quarters – peel the bulbs first if you like. Divide between four plates and transfer a shallot on to each one. Spoon over the cheese. Garnish each plate with extra dill and toasted pumpkin seeds, and drizzle any oil and juices from the foil over the top.

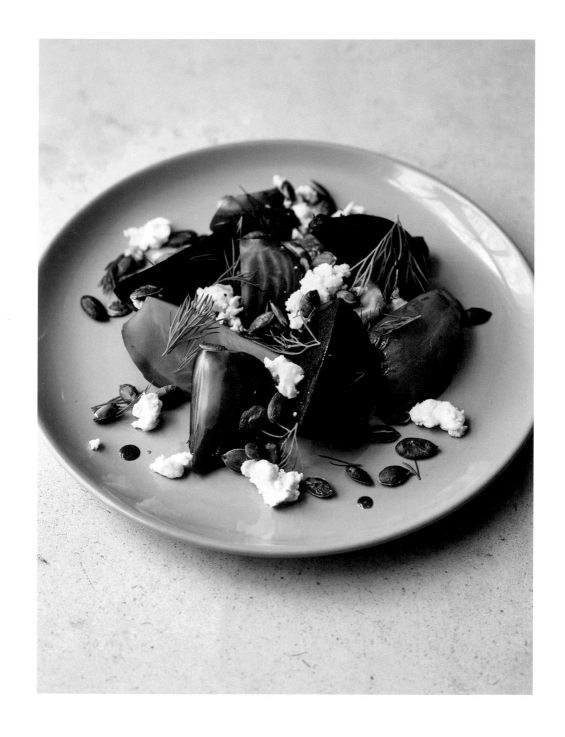

Lettuce Wraps

Forget bread and wrap these yummy fillings in lettuce leaves instead. I find that it's well worth deseeding the cucumber and tomatoes, otherwise the fillings can become very watery.

 SERVES 2   232 calories

For the chicken wraps:

2 iceberg lettuce leaves or 4–5 gem lettuce leaves

2 tsp soy sauce

1 tsp sesame oil

1 tsp sesame seeds

60g leftover cooked roast chicken, shredded

¼ carrot, sliced into matchsticks

2cm piece cucumber, deseeded and sliced into matchsticks

Small handful cress

Freshly ground black pepper

For the hummus wraps:

2 iceberg lettuce leaves or 4–5 gem lettuce leaves

1 tbsp chopped fresh parsley

1 tsp extra virgin olive oil

Zest and juice of 1 lemon

60g hummus

¼ courgette, sliced into matchsticks

¼ red pepper, sliced into matchsticks

2 cherry tomatoes, deseeded and quartered

1 tsp pumpkin seeds

Freshly ground black pepper

- For the chicken wraps, open out the lettuce leaves and put them on a board.

- Put the soy sauce, sesame oil and sesame seeds into a bowl and add the remaining ingredients. Toss well. Spoon the mixture into the lettuce leaves and wrap the leaves around the filling into a parcel. Secure with a cocktail stick. If you're using gem lettuce leaves, divide the mixture evenly between them, and the parcels will be smaller.

- For the hummus wraps, open out the lettuce leaves as before. Put the parsley, oil, and lemon zest and juice in a large bowl and add the hummus, courgette, red pepper, cherry tomatoes and pumpkin seeds. Season, then spoon the filling into the lettuce. Wrap up as before and secure with a cocktail stick.

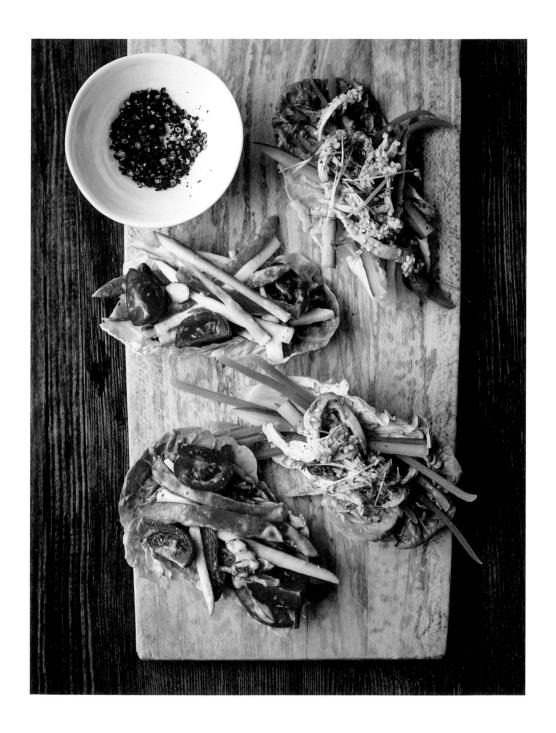

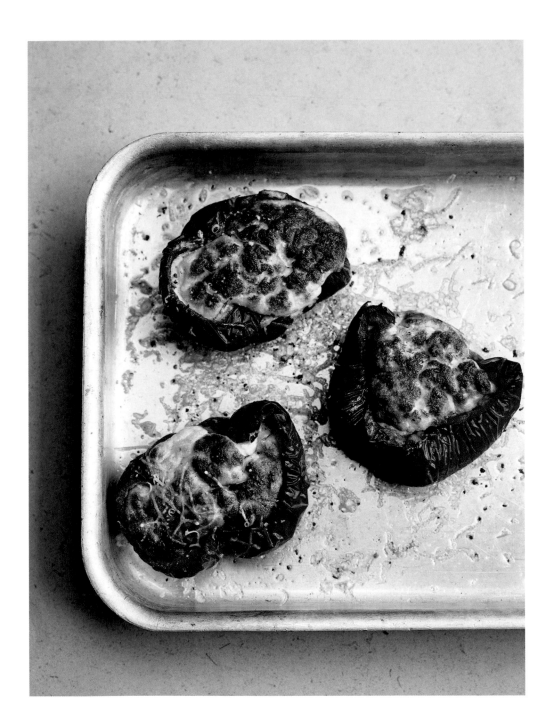

Roast Peppers with Ricotta Soufflé

Roast peppers make perfect little containers for other good things. This soufflé filling is so easy to make and incredibly delicious. My children love this recipe.

GF SERVES 4   290 calories

4 red peppers, halved and deseeded
4 tsp olive oil
4 eggs, separated
200g ricotta
Freshly grated nutmeg
1 tbsp chopped fresh herbs, such as thyme and
   parsley

40g Parmesan, grated
Salt and freshly ground black pepper

To serve:
Steamed green beans and watercress
Lemon wedges

- Preheat the oven to 200°C/400°F/Gas mark 6.

- Lay the pepper halves in a roasting tin. Brush the insides with the oil and season well.

- Put the egg yolks, ricotta, herbs and nutmeg into a bowl with half the Parmesan. Season well and beat together quickly.

- Whisk the egg white in a clean, grease-free bowl until the whites stand in soft peaks. Fold one dessertspoonful into the ricotta mixture to loosen it, then fold in the remainder. Divide evenly between the red pepper halves, then sprinkle with the remaining Parmesan.

- Bake for 15 minutes, until golden. Serve with the green beans and watercress, and a lemon wedge for each person to squeeze over the greens.

MAIN MEALS

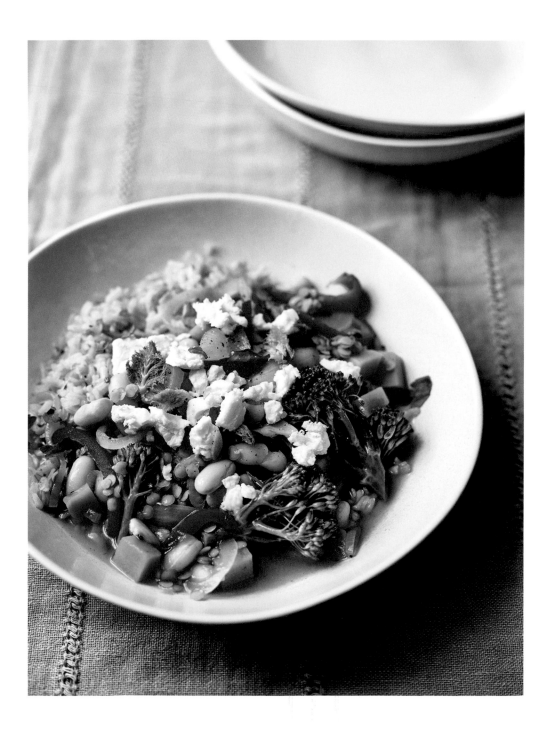

A Bowlful of Goodness

There are so many good things in this recipe – and it tastes great, too. I've kept the amount of rice down, since there are carbs in the beans and lentils, but this is still a really filling, satisfying dish. If you've any leftovers they'll be fine the next day, too.

v   SERVES 4   445 calories

150g short-grain brown rice
2 tbsp olive oil
1 red or white onion, sliced
1 garlic clove, sliced
1 tsp fennel seeds
1 fennel bulb, chopped, fronds reserved
1 red pepper, deseeded and chopped
450g butternut squash, skinned, deseeded
    and chopped
50g red lentils

1 tbsp sundried tomato purée
800ml hot vegetable stock
2 bay leaves
400g can cannellini beans, drained
8 tenderstem broccoli spears
Sea salt and freshly ground black pepper

To serve:
50g feta, crumbled or cut into 4 wedges
2 tbsp chopped fresh parsley

- Put the rice into a saucepan and add 500ml of hot water. Cover with a lid and bring to the boil. Turn the heat down low and simmer for around 25 minutes, until all the water has been absorbed. If the rice is done before everything else, turn the heat off but leave the lid on to keep the rice hot.

- Heat the oil in a large, wide ovenproof pan and cook the onion for 5–10 minutes over a medium heat, until the onion is starting to turn golden. Stir in the garlic and fennel seeds and cook for 1 minute. Season well.

- Add the fennel, pepper, squash and lentils, and give everything a good stir. Allow everything to cook for 5 minutes, stirring every now and then, to soften the vegetables. Whisk the tomato purée into the hot stock, then pour this mixture into the pan. Add the bay leaves and cannellini beans and season again, then cover with a lid and bring to the boil.

- Turn the heat down low and simmer for 20–25 minutes. After 15 minutes, place the broccoli spears on top of the stew and push them just under the top – the heat and remaining liquid will steam them until tender.

- Divide the cooked rice between four bowls and spoon some of the stew over the top, sharing out the broccoli as you go. Place the feta in the middle, scatter the parsley on top, and serve.

Garlic and Ginger Mushrooms with Sprouting Broccoli

This is a great combination of flavours – I always love the tangy taste of fresh root ginger. Broccoli is particularly rich in vitamins and minerals and super-good for our skin.

V DF SERVES 4   284 calories

2 tbsp olive oil

2cm piece of ginger, sliced into matchsticks

2 garlic cloves, sliced

150g shiitake mushrooms, halved

150g chestnut mushrooms, halved, or quartered if large

150g purple sprouting broccoli stems, halved if large

1 tsp sesame seeds

Juice of 1 lime

1 tsp sesame oil

2 tsp soy sauce

1 spring onion, finely sliced

Handful micro herbs, such as basil (optional)

Ground white pepper

For the rice:

5g seaweed

200g short-grain brown rice

400ml hot water

Put the seaweed in a bowl, cover with water and set aside for 15 minutes. Then put the rice into a saucepan, and pour over the hot water. Cover with a lid and bring to the boil. Turn the heat down low and simmer for 20 minutes, until tender, or according to the packet instructions. Drain the seaweed and add to the rice for the last 5 minutes of the cooking time.

Heat the oil in a large wok and add the ginger and garlic. Cook for 1 minute. Add the mushrooms and cook for 5 minutes, until golden. Add the sprouting broccoli and toss everything together. Add 2 tablespoons of water and cover the pan with a lid. The heat will turn the water into steam and help the broccoli to cook until just tender.

Whisk the sesame seeds, lime juice, sesame oil and soy sauce together in a bowl, and season with the white pepper. When the broccoli is tender, pour the dressing over the top of the vegetable mixture.

Divide the rice and seaweed between four bowls, then spoon the stir-fried mushrooms and broccoli over the top. Garnish each bowl with a little spring onion and micro herbs, if using, and serve.

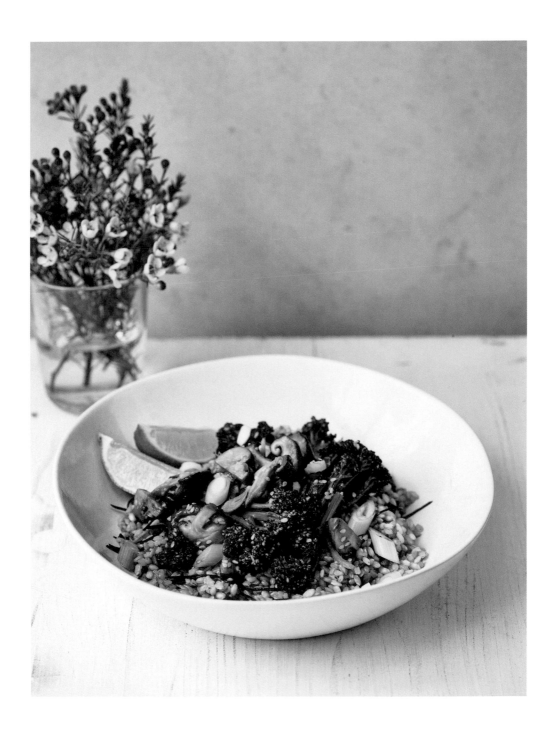

Roasted Vegetables and Butter Beans with Basil Sauce and Toasted Pumpkin Seeds

Enjoy this on its own or alongside some roasted fish or chicken. The vegetables are all cut into quite large chunky pieces and roasting them with the stock keeps them nice and juicy.

V SERVES 4–6 325–217 calories

1 small squash (500g), quartered and deseeded

1 red onion, quartered

2 peppers, halved and deseeded

2 courgettes, halved lengthways

1 aubergine, quartered

2 tbsp olive oil

400ml vegetable stock

400g can butter beans, drained

2 sprigs cherry tomatoes, each loaded with 7–8 tomatoes

3 tbsp Basil Dressing (see page 236)

1 tbsp pumpkin seeds, toasted

Handful rocket, to serve

Sea salt and freshly ground black pepper

- Preheat the oven to 200°C/400°F/Gas mark 6.

- Put the prepared vegetables in a roasting tin. Drizzle the olive oil over the top and toss everything together. Pour in the stock, season and roast for 35–40 minutes.

- Add the butter beans and cherry tomatoes to the tin and return the tin to the oven for 10 minutes, to warm through. Put the Basil Dressing in a small saucepan and heat gently over a very low heat to warm through.

- Divide the vegetables and beans between four to six bowls and drizzle with the sauce, then scatter over the pumpkin seeds and rocket, and serve.

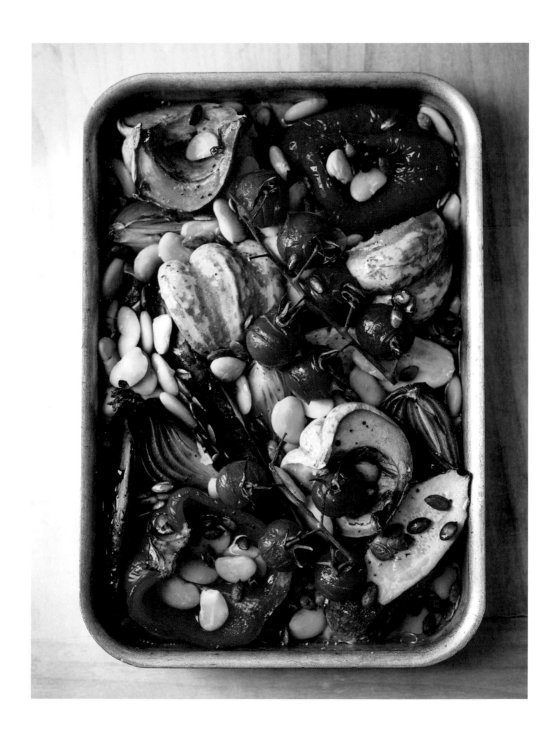

Lentils with Rainbow Vegetables and Kale Pesto

As it stands, this is a delicious vegan feast, but you can add some feta if you like or serve it with some leftover Sunday roast. I love lentils, which are full of healthy fibre and skin-friendly nutrients.

V DF GF   SERVES 4   320 calories

200g puy lentils
2 small beetroot
1 turnip
2 carrots
1 leek
½ head Romanesco cauliflower

½ quantity Kale Pesto (see page 179)
1 tsp mustard seeds
1 tbsp chopped fresh herbs, such as chives,
   parsley or dill

- Put the puy lentils in a saucepan and cover with plenty of water. Cover with a lid and bring to the boil. Turn the heat down low and simmer for 15–20 minutes, until tender.

- Prepare the vegetables: cut the beetroots and turnip into quarters. Chop the carrots on the diagonal into 2.5cm chunks, then do the same with the leek. Break the cauliflower into florets.

- Put all the vegetables in a steamer, or in a pan with 2cm of water. Cover with a lid, then bring to the boil and turn the heat down low. Steam for 10–15 minutes, until tender.

- Make the Kale Pesto (see page 179). If you're making the full quantity, store the remaining amount in a clean jar or sealable container in the fridge for up to 5 days.

- Drain the lentils, stir in the mustard seeds and divide it between four plates. Drain the vegetables and spoon them over the lentils. Put a spoonful of pesto in the middle, then scatter over the herbs. Serve straight away.

Kale Pesto

Kale is very rich in calcium so great for vegans or anyone allergic to dairy products. This pesto keeps well and can be stored in the fridge for up to five days.

V DF GF   MAKES 8 SERVINGS   90 calories

50g kale
6 cherry tomatoes
1 tbsp Dijon mustard

100ml extra virgin olive oil
Juice of ½ lemon
Sea salt and freshly ground black pepper

- Put the kale into a bowl and pour over enough boiling water to cover. Leave for 1 minute, then drain well.

- Transfer the kale to a food processor and add the tomatoes, mustard, oil and lemon juice. Season well. Whizz until smooth. If the mixture is very thick, add 1–2 tablespoons of cold water, to loosen.

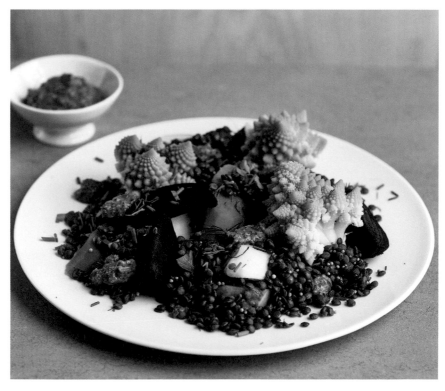

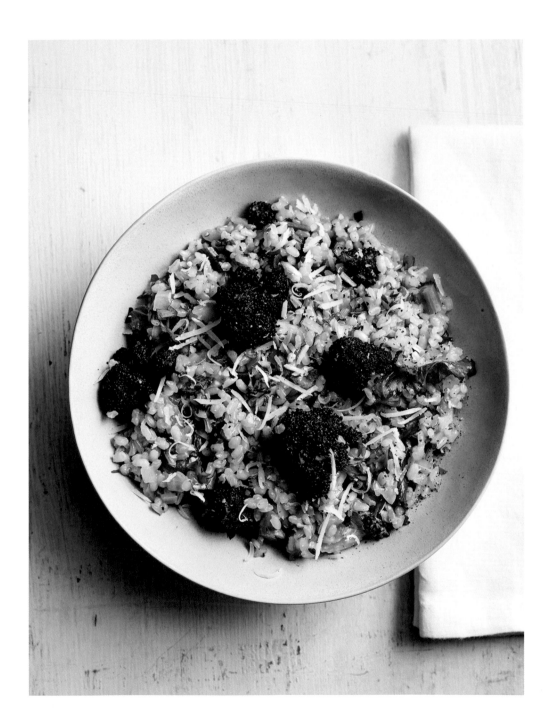

Vegetable risotto

Short-grain brown rice is a great favourite of mine. I love the nutty flavour and I cook it often. I like to use organic rice and I find it's worth buying it in bulk as a store cupboard staple. This risotto works well with sprouting broccoli or asparagus, depending on the season.

v SERVES 4   346 calories

2 tbsp olive oil
1 large banana shallot (or 3 round shallots), finely chopped
1 celery stick, finely chopped
250g short-grain brown rice
1 garlic clove, crushed

1 litre vegetable stock
200g purple sprouting broccoli or asparagus
1 tbsp chopped fresh parsley
25g pecorino cheese (or vegetarian cheese), grated
Sea salt and freshly ground black pepper

- Heat the oil in a pan and add the shallot and celery and 2 tablespoons of water. Season well and stir everything together, then allow the vegetables to cook over a low heat for 5–10 minutes, until softened.

- Stir in the rice and garlic and cook for a minute or two. Stir in the vegetable stock, then put a lid on the pan. Turn the heat down low and allow to simmer for 15 minutes.

- Finely chop the stems of the purple sprouting broccoli or asparagus, leaving the heads/tips with about 1cm of stem on them. After 25 minutes of cooking the rice, stir in the chopped stems and the parsley. Continue to cook for a further 5 minutes with the lid on.

- Stir in the broccoli heads or asparagus tips, then put the lid on and leave to sit for 2–3 minutes. Divide between four bowls and serve with the grated pecorino.

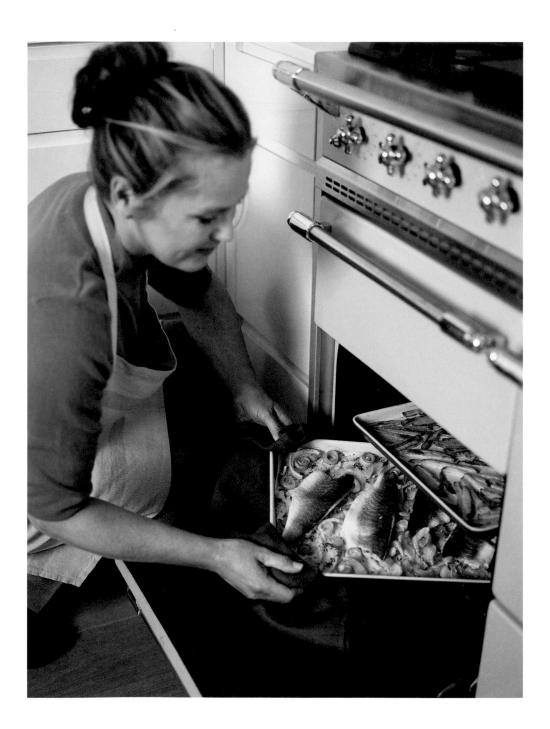

Sea Bass with Leeks, Fennel and Celery

My family calls this 'healthy fish and chips'! It does all have all that lovely yummyness but with lots of extra veggies – and no deep frying. Keep a close eye on the matchstick chips as they near the end of the cooking time so they don't get too dark and burn.

DF SERVES 4   538 calories

2 shallots, finely sliced
2 leeks, finely sliced
1 fennel bulb, finely sliced (reserve the fronds)
2 celery sticks, finely sliced
3 sprigs thyme
3 tbsp olive oil
2–3 large potatoes (around 500g), scrubbed
4 x 175g sea bass fillets

250ml fish, chicken or vegetable stock (see pages 238–239)
Sea salt and freshly ground black pepper

For the dressing:
50g can anchovies in olive oil
1 garlic clove, peeled and sliced
4 tbsp chopped fresh parsley
1 tbsp capers

· Preheat the oven to 200°C/400°F/Gas mark 6. Line a baking sheet with baking parchment.

· Layer the shallots, leeks, fennel, celery and thyme in an ovenproof dish, and season well. Pour over 2 tablespoons of olive oil and mix everything together. Roast in the oven for 10 minutes on the top shelf.

· Cut the potatoes into ½cm slices, then cut each slice into a thin finger. Put the chips in a bowl, toss in the remaining 1 tbsp oil and season well. Spread out on the baking sheet. Pour the stock over the vegetables then transfer to the lower shelf in the oven and put the potato chips on the top shelf. Roast both for 25–30 minutes. Toss the potatoes halfway through the cooking time.

· After 25 minutes, lay the sea bass on top of the vegetables and continue to cook for 10 minutes. Watch the potatoes carefully at this point. If they're golden all over, they're done, so take them out and keep them warm.

· Put the anchovies and the oil from the tin into a small saucepan. Add the garlic and cook for a couple of minutes, until the garlic is golden and the anchovies have broken down. Stir in 1–2 tablespoons water to make a sauce. Take off the heat and stir in the parsley and capers.

· Divide the vegetables and fish between four bowls. Top with the chips, spoon over the anchovy sauce and serve.

Salmon, Fennel and Quinoa Parcels

I love this way of cooking fish – everything is wrapped up neatly in baking parchment and baked in the oven. It's a perfect choice when entertaining friends, as you can get everything ready in advance – see my tip below. To make this dish even more special, you could use red or black quinoa, which looks amazing with the pink fish.

DF SERVES 4   508 calories

1 tbsp olive oil

2 shallots, finely chopped

2 celery sticks, chopped

1 fennel bulb, chopped (reserve the fronds)

1 garlic clove, sliced

200g quinoa

Pinch chilli flakes

500ml hot vegetable stock

2 tbsp chopped fresh parsley

4 salmon fillets

½ lemon, cut into wedges

Sea salt and freshly ground black pepper

- Preheat the oven to 200°C/400°F/Gas mark 6.

- Heat the oil in a pan and sauté the shallots, celery and fennel for 5 minutes, until softened. Stir in the garlic and cook for 1 minute more. Season well. Stir in the quinoa and chilli flakes, then pour over the stock. Cover with a lid and cook for 10 minutes. Stir in the parsley.

- Cut four 30 x 38cm pieces of baking parchment. Spoon a quarter of the quinoa mixture into the middle of each piece of parchment, and put a piece of salmon on top.

- Wrap up one end of each parcel, drizzle 1 tablespoon of water over the salmon and quinoa mixture in each parcel, then wrap up the other end. Put them all on to a baking sheet, then bake in the oven for 15–20 minutes until the fish is cooked. Serve garnished with the reserved fennel fronds and a wedge of lemon.

LIZ'S TIP

If you're making this for a dinner party and want to get ahead, cool the quinoa first before dividing it into the parcels. Once the parcels are made up, put them in the fridge. Take them out half an hour before baking them, so that they're not fridge-cold when they go in the oven.

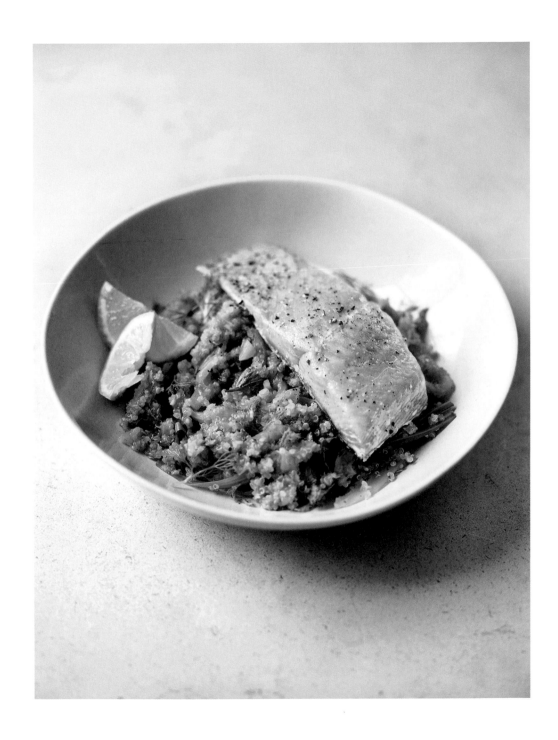

Mackerel with Rice and Rainbow Stir-fry

Cornish mackerel is a sustainable fish and something I cook often. Look for the freshest fish you can find, which should have a lovely glossy blue sheen. I love the flavours of sesame, soy and lime in this dish and you can taste all the individual ingredients.

 SERVES 4   675 calories

5g seaweed
200g short-grain brown rice
4 x 150–175g mackerel fillets
Soy sauce, to season
Sesame oil, to season
1 tbsp toasted sesame seeds

For the rainbow stir-fry:
2 tbsp rapeseed oil
1 red onion, finely sliced

1 large carrot, cut into batons
10 cavolo nero leaves, finely chopped
1 yellow pepper, halved, deseeded and
   finely sliced
1 fat garlic clove, finely sliced
2.5cm piece fresh root ginger, cut into matchsticks
1 tsp sesame oil
1 lime, cut into wedges, to serve
Ground white pepper

- Put the seaweed in a bowl, cover with cold water and set aside. Put the brown rice into a saucepan and pour over 500ml of cold water. Cover with a lid and bring to the boil. Turn the heat down low and simmer for 25–30 minutes. The water will be absorbed, and the rice should still have a tender bite. About 15 minutes before the rice has finished cooking, preheat the grill.

- Heat the oil in a large wok or frying pan and add the onion, carrot, cavolo nero and pepper. Cook for 2–3 minutes until they are starting to soften, then add the garlic and ginger and cook for 1 minute more. Add 2 tablespoons of water and toss everything together. Season with the pepper and cover with a lid so that the vegetables steam in the pan.

- Brush the flesh side of the mackerel fillets with soy sauce then with the sesame oil, and grill for 5–10 minutes until the fish is cooked through.

- Drain the seaweed and put it on top of the rice. Add sesame oil to the stir-fry and toss everything together. Divide the rice mixture and the vegetables between four plates. Top with a mackerel fillet and serve sprinkled with the sesame seeds and the lime wedges.

LIZ'S TIP

Sardines work well in this recipe, too. Ask your fishmonger to remove the bones, and serve two per person.

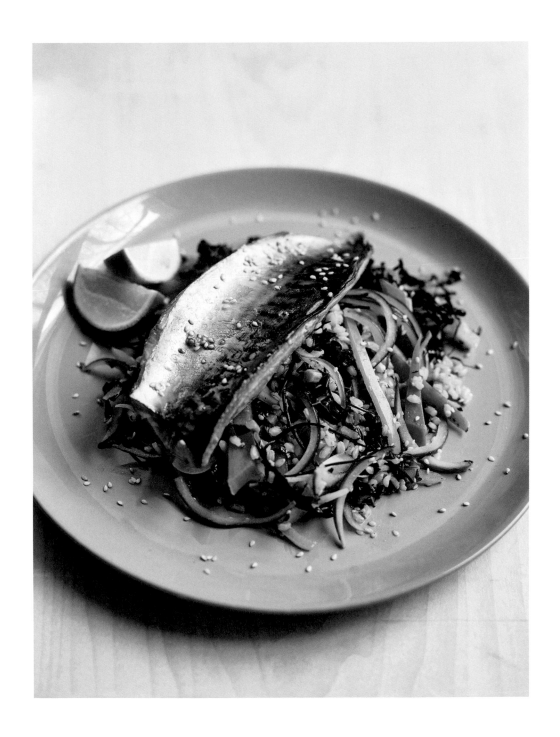

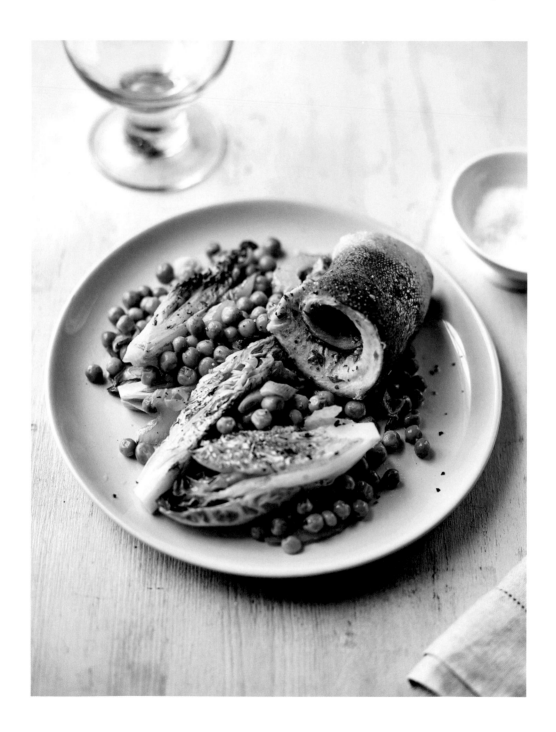

Pink Trout with Buttered Lettuce

Oily fish, like trout, salmon and mackerel, is packed with Omega-3 and so is really good for our skin. In this recipe the trout fillets are spinkled with lots of fresh herbs, then rolled up neatly for cooking. You can secure each roll with a cocktail stick if you like, but I find they hold together well once the fish starts cooking.

GF SERVES 4   254 calories

4 trout fillets, with skin, pin-boned   4 spring onions, sliced
4 anchovy fillets   1 celery stick, finely sliced
1 tbsp chopped fresh tarragon   2 gem lettuces, quartered lengthways
2 tbsp chopped fresh parsley   10g butter
1 tbsp rapeseed or olive oil   150g frozen peas, thawed
                                               Sea salt and freshly ground black pepper

- Lay the trout on a board skin side down, and put an anchovy fillet into the middle of each. Sprinkle each fillet with a good pinch of the herbs (around half in total) and season well.

- Roll up the fish from the tail end, keeping the seam tucked underneath. Skewer with a cocktail stick if you think the filets need to be secured.

- Heat the oil in a large frying pan and gently sauté the spring onions and celery for 5–10 minutes, until soft. Increase the heat a little and put the lettuce quarters, flat-side down, in the pan. Turn them over once they're golden.

- Heat a separate pan – a wok is ideal for this – and add the trout, seam-side down. There should be no need for any oil. Add 1–2 tablespoons of water to the pan, cover with a lid and cook for 8–10 minutes, until the fish is opaque.

- Add the butter, peas and 2 tablespoons of water to the pan containing the lettuce, and season well. Cover with a lid and cook for 3–4 minutes over a low heat. Scatter over the remaining herbs.

- Put a trout roll on each plate, and spoon the buttered lettuce and peas alongside. Drizzle any juices left in each pan over the top.

Healthy Fish Pie

This pie makes a welcome change from the usual creamy versions and my kids absolutely love it. In fact, I always make extra to stash in the freezer, ready for a quick supper on extra-busy nights. The scallops are a treat but you can just use white fish for a more economical meal.

SERVES 4   326 calories

1 tbsp olive oil

2 shallots, finely chopped

2 celery sticks, finely chopped

1 red pepper, halved, deseeded and chopped

1 garlic clove, finely sliced

350g passata rustica

1 tsp paprika

1 tbsp sundried tomato purée

250ml hot fish, chicken or vegetable stock

2 tbsp chopped fresh parsley

4 green queen olives, stoned and chopped

75g sourdough bread

700g white fish fillet, such as pollock, cut into 2.5cm squares

4 scallops with roe, separated and trimmed

60g Gruyère cheese, grated

Sea salt and freshly ground black pepper

- Heat the oil in a pan and sauté the shallots and celery over a low to medium heat for 5 minutes, until softened. Stir in the pepper and garlic and continue to cook for a further 5 minutes.

- Stir in the passata, paprika, sundried tomato purée and stock. Season well. Cover the pan with a lid and bring to the boil, then reduce the heat and simmer for 20 minutes until slightly reduced. Stir in the parsley and olives.

- Preheat the oven to 200°C/400°F/Gas mark 6. Whizz the sourdough bread into breadcrumbs in a small food processor. Put the fish into a 1.5–2 litre ovenproof dish or divide it between four 450ml pie dishes, placing a scallop in the middle of each. Season, then pour over the sauce. Scatter the breadcrumbs over the sauce, then top with the Gruyère.

- For one pie, bake for around 30–40 minutes or 25–35 minutes for individual pies, making sure the fish is cooked through and the pie is bubbling hot.

LIZ'S TIP

To prepare ahead, make the sauce to the end of the second step and chill for up to three days, or freeze for up to 1 month. Store the fish and toppings in separate freezer-proof containers, then thaw everything overnight at room temperature, or in the fridge. Once thawed, put everything together as above.

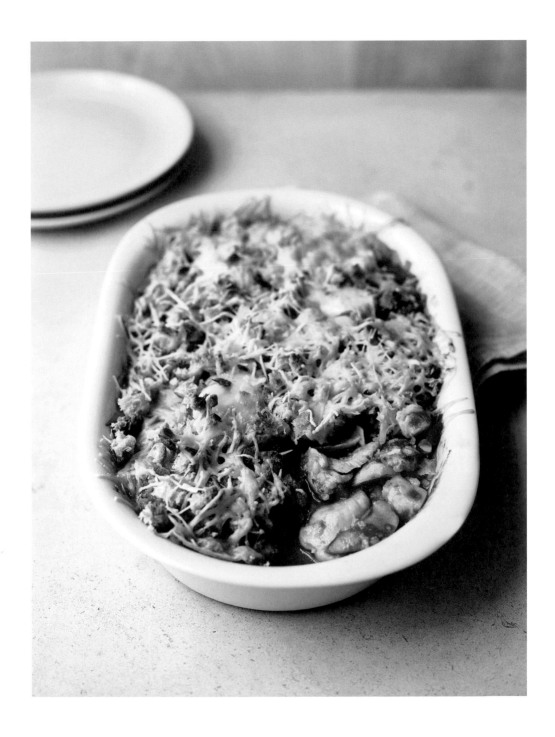

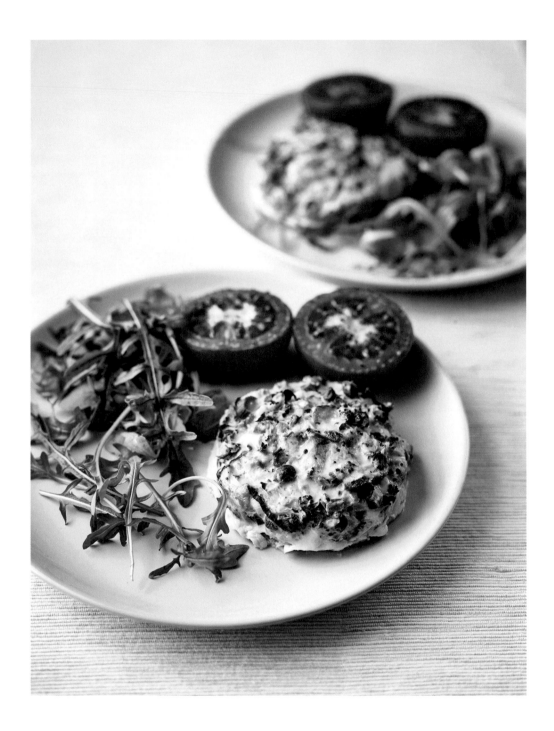

Salmon Fishcakes

Most fishcakes are heavy with potato but these are much lighter – and very good. Easy to make, but you do need to chop the salmon and the broccoli into nice small pieces so that the mixture holds together when packed into the cutter.

GF   SERVES 4   256 calories

4 spears purple sprouting broccoli, very finely
    chopped
1 shallot, very finely chopped
2 x 150g salmon fillets, without skin
1–2 tbsp beaten egg
30g pecorino, grated
2 gherkins, very finely chopped

1 tsp nonpareille capers
5g chives, finely chopped
Sea salt and freshly ground black pepper

To serve:
4 tomatoes, halved
Handful of rocket

- Preheat the oven to 200°C/400°F/Gas mark 6. Line a baking sheet with baking parchment.

- Put the broccoli and shallot in a bowl. Pour enough boiling water over them to cover, and set aside for 2–3 minutes.

- Chop the salmon into ½cm pieces and put it in a bowl with the beaten egg, pecorino, gherkins, capers and chives. Drain the broccoli very well until no excess water remains – otherwise the fishcakes might not stay together. Stir into the salmon mixture and season well.

- Put an 8cm round cutter on to the baking sheet and spoon a quarter of the mixture into it, pressing the mixture down to compress it slightly. Lift up the cutter and do the same again to make four fishcakes.

- Put two halves of tomato next to each fishcake, and season well. Transfer to the oven and bake for 15–20 minutes, until the fish is cooked through.

- Transfer a fishcake to each plate, and serve with the tomatoes and rocket.

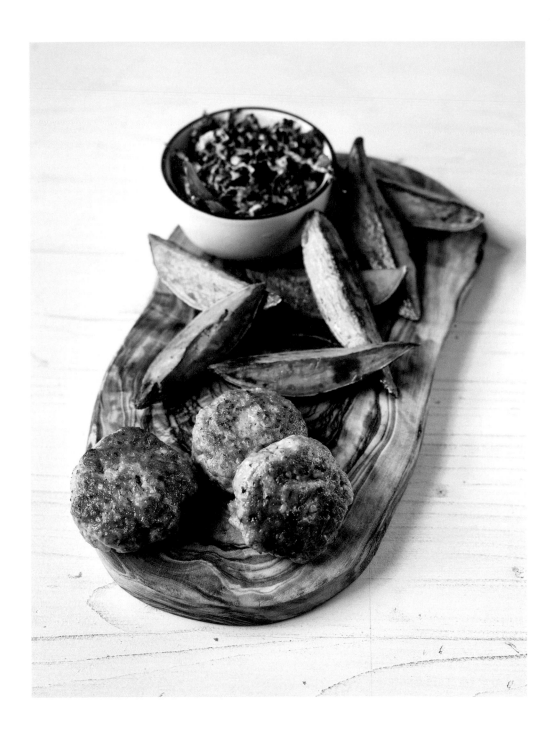

Spicy Chicken Burgers with Sweet Potato Wedges

Here's my skin-friendly version of burger and chips! The cayenne in the burger mix does give quite a kick so if you're not a fan of spicy heat, just use a pinch or half a teaspoonful. My family like the mini burgers but you can make them larger if you like and just cook them for longer. I love the sweet potato wedges, too and you can cook them on top of the stove with only a smidgen of oil.

GF SERVES 4   390 calories

500g skinless, boneless chicken thighs or breasts
2 shallots or ¼ red onion, finely chopped
½–1 tsp cayenne pepper
1 tsp ground coriander
1 tsp fresh or dried thyme
1 tbsp olive or rapeseed oil
2 medium sweet potatoes, quartered
Sea salt and freshly ground black pepper

For the salad:
1 red pepper, finely sliced
4 cavolo nero leaves, finely sliced
1 small kohlrabi, peeled and cut into matchsticks

For the dressing:
½ quantity Mustard Dressing (see page 237)
2 tsp Greek yoghurt

- Put the chicken, shallots or red onion, cayenne pepper, coriander and thyme into a food processor, and season well. Blend to mince the chicken and make a smooth mixture. Spoon the mixture into a bowl.

- Wet your hands and divide the mixture into four parts. Divide one of these parts into three, and shape each piece into a mini burger. Place them on a board. Do the same with the rest of the mixture until you've made 12 burgers. Set aside just while you start to cook the sweet potatoes. The burgers will be fine at room temperature, and it allows all the ingredients to come together.

- Heat ½ tablespoon of oil in a large frying pan, and place the sweet potato wedges flat-side down in the pan. Cook for 1–2 minutes until golden. Flip to the other flat side and do the same again. Add about 3 tablespoons of water to the pan, season well and cover with a lid, and cook for around 20 minutes, until the potato is tender and cooked through.

- Heat the remaining oil in a separate large frying pan and fry the burgers until cooked through and golden on each side – this will take around 8 minutes in total.

- Make the Mustard Dressing, then put half of it in a bowl. Stir in the yoghurt. Add the salad ingredients, season and toss everything together. Divide the sweet potato wedges between four plates. Add the burgers and serve with the salad.

Roast Lemon Chicken with Spring Vegetables

If you can, it's well worth buying organic chicken for its superb taste as well as the animal welfare concerns. The flavour of a properly reared bird is incomparable and adds another dimension to the sauce in this dish. The lemons are amazing too, as they roast until they are beautifully soft and jammy and they can be served with the chicken and vegetables.

SERVES 4, WITH PLENTY OF LEFTOVER CHICKEN 395 calories

1 large onion, sliced

2 lemons, halved

2–3 sprigs rosemary

1 fresh chicken, around 2.5kg

750ml chicken or vegetable stock (see page 238)

1 tbsp olive oil

Sea salt and freshly ground black pepper

For the vegetables and herb butter:

100g asparagus tips, trimmed

75g green beans, trimmed

75g mangetout

75g peas

100g baby courgettes, halved lengthways

15g Herb Butter (see page 207)

- Preheat the oven to 200°C/400°F/Gas mark 6. Calculate the cooking time for the chicken, working on the basis of 20 minutes per 500g, plus 20 minutes.

- Place the onion in the base of a roasting tin and place a lemon half in each corner of the tin. Push the rosemary into the chicken and place the chicken on top of the onions. Pour the stock into the tin. Drizzle the olive oil on top, season, and cover the whole tin with foil. Transfer to the oven and cook for 1 hour.

- Remove the foil and continue to cook the chicken for the remaining time (around 1 hour). To check the chicken is cooked, pierce the thigh with a skewer – it's ready when the juices run clear and no pink juices remain. Take the chicken out of the oven, transfer it to a warm platter and cover it with a clean sheet of foil. Set aside to rest for 10 minutes.

- Bring a large pan of water to the boil and add the asparagus, beans, mangetout, peas and baby courgettes. Cover and simmer for 4–5 minutes until the vegetables are tender. Drain well. Return to the pan, add the Herb Butter and season, then cover with the lid to keep warm.

- While the vegetables are cooking, pour the sauce from the chicken into a large jug. The onions will fall to the bottom and the fat will rise to the top. Skim off and discard as much of the fat as possible. To serve, slice the chicken, spoon over some of the sauce and give everyone a lemon half, and serve with the vegetables.

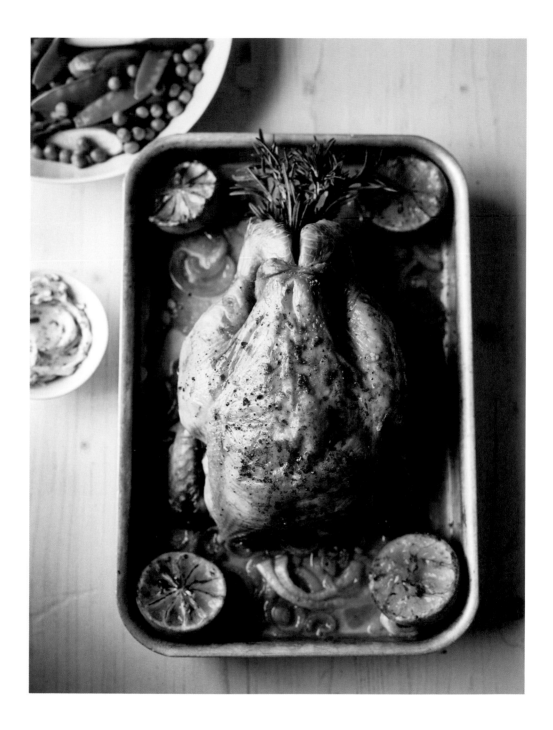

A Simple Chicken Supper

With good free-range or organic chicken the flavour of this simple dish will be great and you'll have a really tasty sauce. Do be sure to serve the garlic cloves, which will be soft and delicious by the end of the cooking time.

 SERVES 4   395 calories

1 tbsp olive or rapeseed oil

4 chicken breasts, skin on, each around 150g

4 garlic cloves, unpeeled

6 spring onions, chopped into 1.5cm pieces

½ lime, cut into 4 wedges

150ml water

Sea salt and freshly ground black pepper

For the broccoli and sugarsnaps:

1 quantity of Pumpkin Seed Dressing (see page 236)

250g broccoli, cut into florets

125g sugarsnaps or fresh peas

8 radishes, halved

- Heat the oil in a large frying pan. Season the chicken well then place each piece skin-side down in the pan, and fry for 2–3 minutes until golden. Turn over to brown the other side.

- Add the garlic, chopped spring onion and lime to the pan and pour in the water. Put a lid on the pan, allow the liquid to start simmering, then turn the heat down to low and cook for 10 minutes.

- Take the lid off the pan and continue to simmer for around 5 minutes more, until the liquid has reduced to a sauce and the chicken is cooked through.

- Meanwhile, make the Pumpkin Seed Dressing (see page 236), adding the water according to the instructions.

- Bring a medium pan of water to the boil and add the broccoli florets. Allow to cook for 1 minute, then add the sugarsnaps. Cook for around 3 minutes more, until the broccoli is tender. If you're using peas, cook the broccoli for 2 minutes first.

- Just before draining the vegetables, add the radish halves to the pan to warm through. Drain well, then return the vegetables to the pan and add the dressing, tossing well.

- Divide the chicken, garlic and spring onion between four plates, then divide the vegetables between the plates, too. Spoon the sauce over the chicken, and serve.

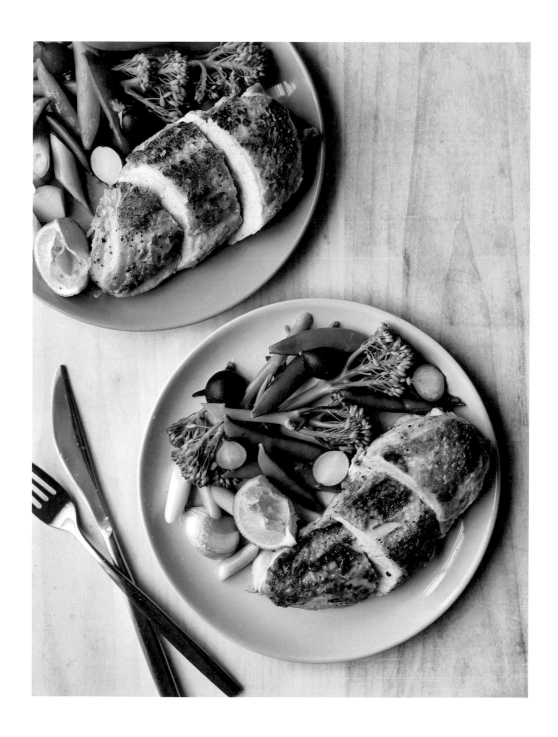

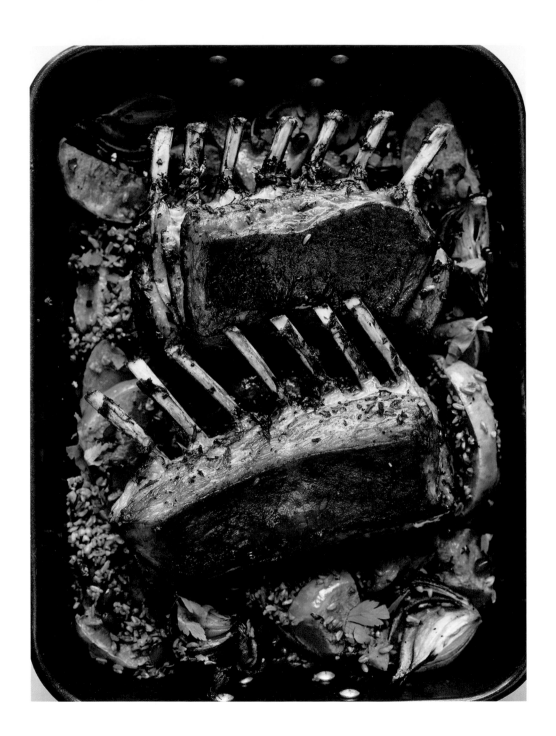

Rack of Lamb with Freekeh and Roasted Squash

I make this often for family and friends. Rack of lamb is always good to eat and if you marinate the racks for eight hours they taste even better. Freekeh is harvested as a green grain, which is then roasted or smoked, giving it a deliciously nutty flavour.

 SERVES 4   521 calories

2 racks of lamb, each with 7–8 cutlets
1 sprig rosemary, chopped
Small handful parsley, roughly chopped
Small handful thyme leaves, chopped
1 garlic clove, sliced
125ml red wine
1 red onion, cut into 4 wedges
½ small butternut squash, peeled, deseeded and
   cut into small wedges

2 tbsp olive oil
100g freekeh
200ml chicken or vegetable stock
Seeds of ½ pomegranate
Small handful parsley, finely chopped
Sea salt and freshly ground black pepper

- Up to 8 hours ahead, put the racks of lamb in a sealable container and add the rosemary, parsley, thyme, garlic and red wine. Cover and transfer to the fridge to marinate.

- When you're ready to cook the lamb, take it out of the fridge to let it come up to room temperature. Preheat the oven to 200°C/400°F/Gas mark 6. Put the red onion and squash in a roasting tin, drizzle over the oil and season well. Roast in the oven for 20 minutes.

- Put the freekeh in a large saucepan and cover with 500ml of boiling water. Cover, bring to the boil and then reduce the heat to a simmer and cook for 15 minutes. Meanwhile, heat a large frying pan until hot. Lift the lamb out of the marinade and scrape off any herbs. Season it well and fry the racks of lamb, skin-side down, until golden.

- Reduce the temperature of the oven to 180°C/350°F/Gas mark 4. Transfer the racks to the roasting tin and continue to cook for a further 20–25 minutes, depending on their thickness.

- Put the racks on a warm plate, cover with foil and leave to rest. Strain the marinade into a pan and add the stock. Bring to a simmer and cook until reduced by half. Taste to make sure it's seasoned properly.

- Stir the freekeh, pomegranate seeds and parsley into the roasted vegetables. Divide between four plates. Slice the racks, giving each person 3–4 cutlets each, and drizzle with the sauce.

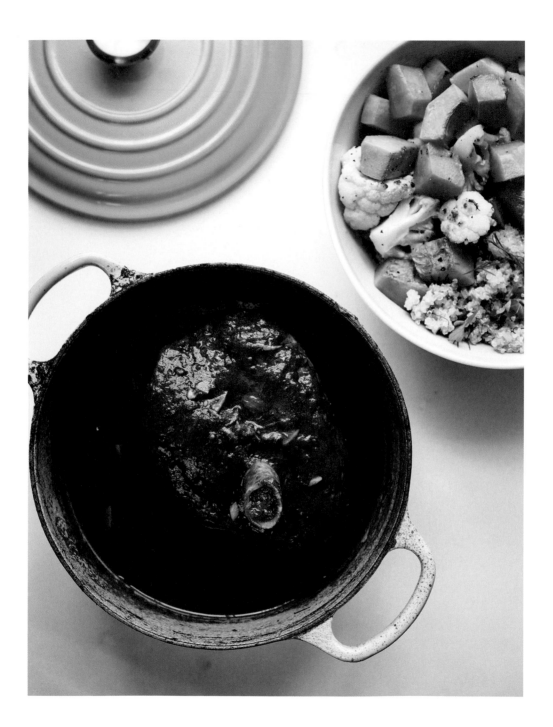

Leg of Lamb with an Instant Sauce

Lamb is my favourite meat and this recipe is so easy to do. You just pop the joint in the oven and leave it to cook to melting tenderness. The juices in the dish provide a wonderful sauce.

DF **SERVES 4, WITH LEFTOVERS**   564 calories

For the lamb:
1 onion, chopped
4 garlic cloves, unpeeled
100ml red wine
550ml chicken or vegetable stock
175g passata rustica
1.25kg leg of lamb
Sea salt and freshly ground black pepper

For the quinoa, squash and cauliflower:
½ butternut squash, peeled, deseeded and cut into
   3cm cubes
½ cauliflower, broken into florets
1 tbsp olive oil
1–2 pinches chilli powder
200g quinoa
500ml hot vegetable stock
2 tbsp chopped fresh parsley
2 tbsp chopped fresh dill
1 tbsp chopped fresh mint

- Preheat the oven to 180°C/350°F/Gas mark 4. Put the onion and garlic in a medium casserole or roasting tin. Add the wine, stock and passata, and season well. Stir everything together. Place the lamb in the dish too, then cover. Transfer the tin to the oven and cook for 4 hours.

- About 45 minutes before the end of the cooking time, mix the squash, cauliflower, olive oil and chilli powder in a bowl. Scoop out the squash and put it in a roasting tin with 1 tablespoon of water, then cook with the lamb. After 15 minutes, add the cauliflower to the squash in the tin and add another tablespoon of water. Cook for a further 20–25 minutes, until the squash is tender.

- About 15 minutes before the lamb is ready, put the quinoa in a saucepan and add the stock. Cover with a lid and bring to the boil over a high heat. Turn the heat down low and simmer until all the liquid has been absorbed and the quinoa has cooked.

- Once the lamb is cooked, take it out of the oven, leaving the lid or foil on, and set aside to rest for 10 minutes. Add the herbs to the quinoa, and season well. Spoon the quinoa into a bowl and top with the roasted vegetables. Carve the lamb, and serve it with the sauce and the quinoa.

LIZ'S TIP

For a pull-apart shredded joint, use shoulder of lamb (same weight). Follow the method and timings, then before serving set the roasting tin aside to rest for 5 minutes. Carefully drain the fat off, then pull the meat apart and serve with the sauce.

Lamb Kebabs with Tabbouleh

Who doesn't love a kebab? I serve mine with this special tabbouleh. It's made with some blitzed cauliflower as well as bulgar wheat and so upping the veg content and cutting the carb count.

 SERVES 4 360 calories

500g lean lamb leg or shoulder, cut into
   3cm cubes
1 tsp olive oil
sprig of rosemary
1 tsp paprika
Sea salt and freshly ground black pepper

For the tabbouleh:
¼ cauliflower, roughly chopped
100g bulgar wheat
200ml hot chicken or vegetable stock
2 large tomatoes, halved and deseeded
¼ cucumber
1 orange or yellow pepper, halved and deseeded
20g parsley, finely chopped
10g chives, finely chopped
1 tbsp olive oil
Zest and juice of ½ lemon

- Put the lamb into a bowl and add the oil, rosemary and paprika. Season well and toss everything together. Set aside for at least 30 minutes. (You can marinate it overnight, too.) Soak four wooden skewers in a bowl of cold water.

- Put the cauliflower into a food processor and whizz until it is finely blitzed. Put it in a large bowl with the bulgar wheat and pour over the hot stock. Season well and set aside to soak for around 20 minutes.

- Preheat the grill and push the lamb on to the skewers. Grill for 15–20 minutes, turning halfway through, until the cubes are cooked but still pink inside.

- When the bulghur mixture has finished soaking, prepare the other vegetables. Chop the tomatoes finely and put into the bowl with the bulghur. Do the same with the cucumber, deseeding it first if you prefer, and the pepper. Add the parsely and chives to the bowl with the oil, lemon zest and juice. Season well and stir everything together. Divide between four plates and top each portion of tabbouleh with a lamb skewer.

LIZ'S TIP

You can also serve the skewers in flatbreads. Finely shred 1 gem lettuce and divide between 4 small wholemeal pitta breads or flatbreads. Spoon over 1 tablespoon tabbouleh, and top with the skewers.

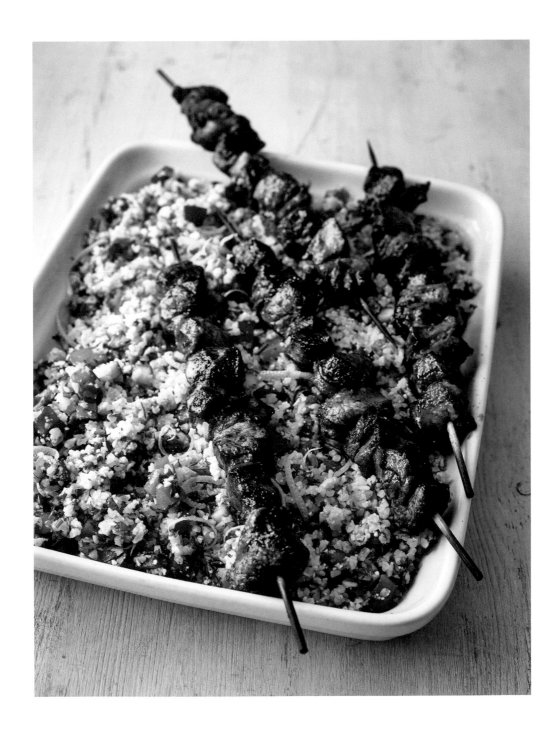

Healthy, Nourishing Steak

This recipe is a great way of making two good steaks stretch to four people, by serving them with lots of veggies. Grilling the vegetables gives them a good texture, but do watch them closely so they don't burn. This steak is delicious served with the herb butter on the page opposite, but leave this out if you are dairy-free.

DF GF **SERVES 4**   **300 calories**

1 tsp oil

2 tsp chopped fresh woody herbs
(such as rosemary and thyme)

2 sirloin steaks with a thin rim of fat
(around 500g in total)

Small handful basil, roughly torn, to garnish

For the vegetables:

2 tsp olive oil

2 baby cauliflowers, trimmed and quartered

1 red onion, halved and each half cut into 4 wedges

4 plum tomatoes, halved

150g green beans, halved

50g watercress or rocket

Salt and freshly ground black pepper

For the dressing:

1 tbsp extra virgin olive oil

1 tbsp balsamic vinegar or 2 tbsp
Basil Dressing (see page 236)

- Preheat the grill. Put the oil and herbs into a shallow dish, and mix together. Add the steaks, then flip each steak over so they're both covered in the mixture. Set aside to marinate. You can do this up to 4 hours ahead, but store the steak in the fridge and take it out about 30 minutes before you're ready to cook it.

- For the veg, brush the oil over the cauliflower, red onion and plum tomatoes, and season well. Put them on a baking sheet and grill for 15–20 minutes, until golden. Flip the onions over halfway through, and turn the cauliflower around, too. Watch carefully to ensure the pieces don't burn.

- Heat a large frying pan over a medium heat until hot. Season the steaks and fry them for 3–5 minutes on each side, until cooked medium. Meanwhile, cook the green beans in a saucepan of boiling water for 3–4 minutes, until tender. Drain well. Arrange the watercress over a large platter.

- When the steaks are ready, set aside on a warm plate to rest. Add the olive oil and vinegar to the pan with 1 tablespoon of water. Stir together, ensuring that the juices from the pan dissolve, too. Add any juices from resting the steaks, then take the pan off the heat.

- Scatter the beans and grilled vegetables over the rocket and basil. Slice the steak into thin slivers then arrange them over the top. Spoon the dressing all over and serve. Alternatively, cut each steak in half and serve with the vegetables and a serving of herb butter (right) with each half.

Herb Butter

This butter goes perfectly with my steak recipe on the page opposite. It's well worth keeping some of this butter in the freezer – it keeps for a couple of months.

GF V   MAKES 150G/10 SERVINGS   77 calories

100g salted butter, at room temperature
10g chopped fresh chives
10g chopped fresh parsley
5g chopped fresh dill

1 tbsp Dijon or grainy mustard
Good grind black pepper
Good pinch cayenne pepper

Put the butter in a bowl, and beat to soften. Add the herbs, mustard, black pepper and cayenne, and mix again. Scrape the mixture out of the bowl and put it into a piece of baking parchment. Wrap well, shaping it into a barrel shape. Chill until firm.

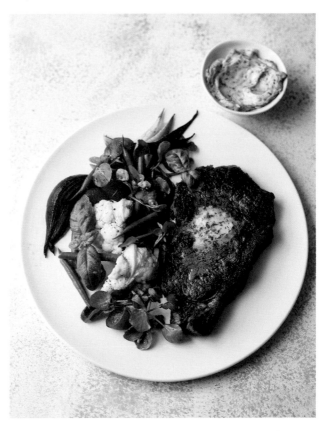

DESSERTS AND TREATS

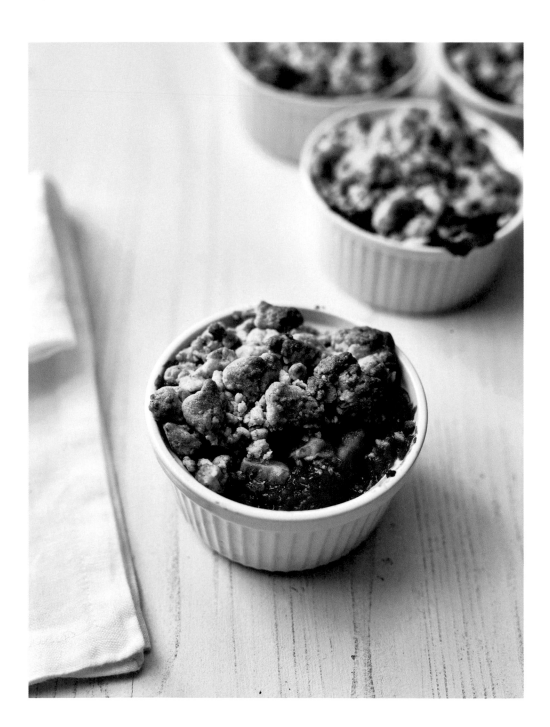

Raspberry and Apple Crisp

These little puddings might look dainty but the oats and nuts in the topping help to make them surprisingly filling. Lovely with a spoonful of Greek yoghurt on top if you fancy.

v SERVES 4   216 calories

For the topping:
30g butter
30g set honey
35g wholemeal or spelt flour
15g jumbo oats
15g walnuts

For the filling:
1 medium Bramley apple
Juice of ½ orange
½ tsp ground cinnamon
2 tsp honey or maple syrup
150g raspberries

- Preheat the oven to 190°C/375°F/Gas mark 5.

- Peel, core and finely chop the apple, put it in a bowl with the orange juice and mix well. Add the cinnamon, honey or maple syrup and raspberries, and stir everything together. Divide this mixture between four 150ml ramekins. It will almost fill the ramekins, but don't worry as the fruit cooks down during baking.

- Put all the ingredients for the topping into a mini food processor. Pulse to chop the oats and walnuts, until the mixture looks like a very rough crumble.

- Spoon the topping evenly between the ramekins. You may need to pile the mixture up so it looks like a bit of a tower, but as it bakes it will cook down. Transfer to a baking sheet and bake in the oven for 20–25 minutes, until the fruit is soft and the top is crisp – hence the name!

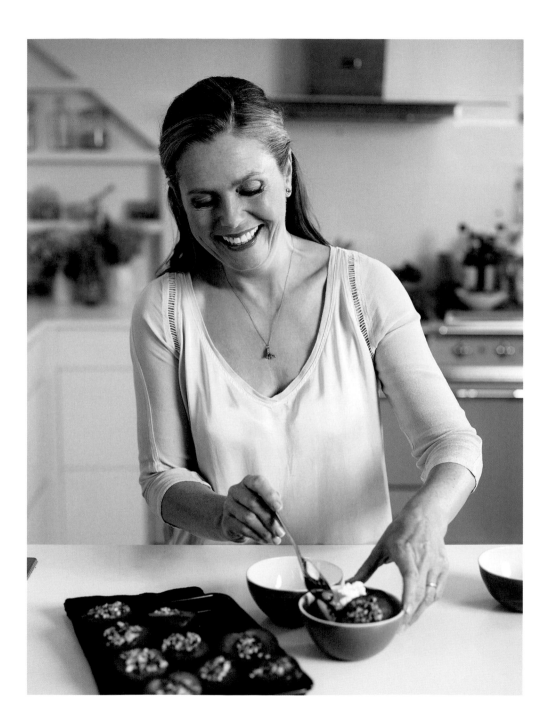

Grilled Plums

Plums, spice and almonds are perfect partners and this pudding is super quick to put together. If you're using the big bubblegum plums, six should be plenty, but when Victoria plums are in season, you'll probably need eight, so everyone can have four halves. Enjoy the plums as they are or serve them with a spoonful of ricotta on the side.

V GF SERVES 4   121 calories

6–8 plums, depending on size
15g softened unsalted butter
1 tsp set honey
20g whole almonds, finely chopped
¼ tsp mixed spice

To serve:
4 tbsp ricotta (optional)

- Preheat the grill to hot. While it's heating up, cut the plums in half and take out the stones.

- Beat the butter and honey together in a bowl, then fold in the almonds and mixed spice. Spoon evenly between the plum halves. It won't look like much, but the butter melts into the fruit as it cooks and is there to season the fruit, not to overpower it.

- Transfer the plums to a baking sheet and grill for 5–6 minutes until golden and bubbling. Serve straight away with the ricotta, if using.

Rich Chocolate Pots

I love dark chocolate and luckily research shows that it's good for us and skin – in small amounts obviously! These little pots are rich and very satisfying.

V GF SERVES 4 117 calories

5 dried prunes, stoned and chopped
60ml apple juice
¼ tsp ground cinnamon
1 tsp vanilla extract

50g dark chocolate (minimum 80% cocoa solids)
1 egg, separated

To serve:
4 tsp Greek yoghurt

- Put the prunes and apple juice into a small saucepan with the cinnamon and vanilla extract. Bring to the boil, then set aside to soak for 30 minutes.

- Melt the chocolate in a bowl resting over a pan of boiling water, making sure the base doesn't touch the water. Set aside to cool a little. Alternatively, you can put the chocolate in a bowl and melt it in the microwave on low.

- Whizz the prune mixture in a blender until smooth, then strain through a sieve into a bowl to extract a smooth purée. Stir the egg yolk into the prune purée, then carefully stir in the melted chocolate.

- Whisk the egg white in a spotlessly clean, grease-free bowl until soft peaks form. Fold a large spoonful of egg white into the prune mixture, then carefully fold in the rest, taking care not to knock too much air out.

- Spoon the mixture between four little pots (each measuring 60ml) and chill for 30 minutes, or up to 1 hour. When you're ready to serve, finish each pot with a spoonful of yoghurt on top.

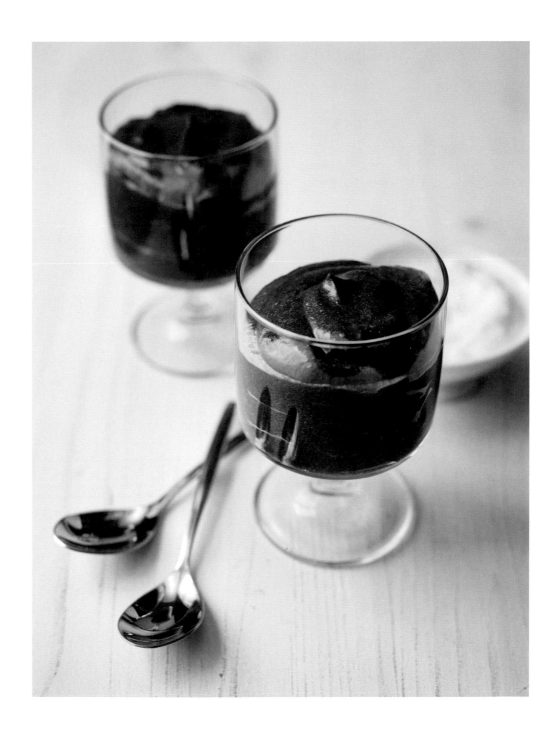

Cinnamon Poached Pears

Pears are a good source of potassium, phosphorus and calcium as well as vitamins C and B. These poached pears, with a touch of citrus, cinnamon and star anise, make a perfect sweet finish to a meal. This is one of my favourite puddings.

V DF GF   SERVES 4   100 calories

4 firm pears

1 tbsp honey or maple syrup

Juice of 2 oranges

1 cinnamon stick

Strip orange peel

1 star anise

- Peel the pears and remove the calyx at the bottom using a sharp knife.

- Put them in a pan just large enough so that they fit snugly against each other. Add the honey or maple syrup, orange juice, cinnamon stick, orange peel and star anise. Pour in enough cold water for the liquid to come about three-quarters up the pears.

- Cut a piece of baking parchment to fit the top of the pan, then scrunch it up and open it out again so it's all crumpled. Fit it over the pears so it's touching them. Cover the pan with a lid and bring it to the boil, then turn the heat down low and simmer for 15 minutes. Turn the pears over, then simmer again for another 10 minutes until tender and you can push a knife all the way to the centre.

- Leave the pears to marinate in the liquid. When you're ready to serve, take the pears out of the pan and set them aside. Lift out and discard the cinnamon stick, orange peel and star anise. Bring the liquid to the boil and simmer, without a lid, for about 5 minutes until it has reduced and is syrupy. Serve spooned over the pears.

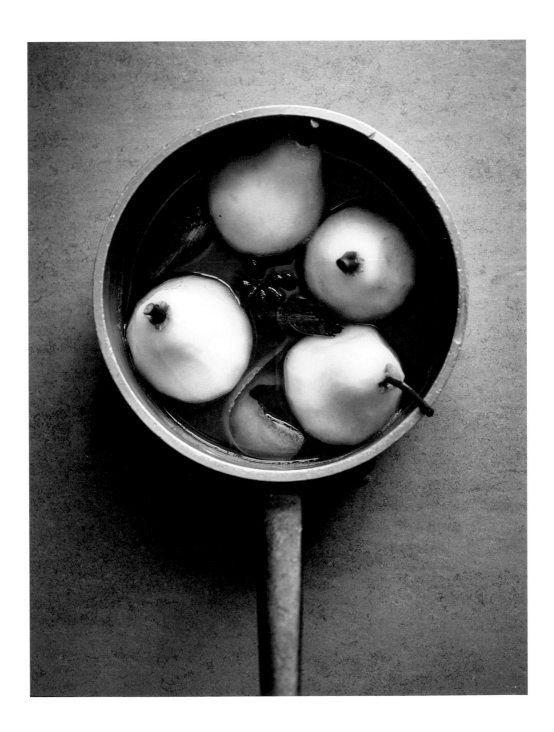

Blackberry, Hazelnut and Spelt Cake Bites

There is a small amount of honey in these delicious little bars but no refined sugar. Most of the sweetness comes from the fresh and dried fruit. Well wrapped, these keep well for about five days or you can pop some in the freezer for another time. They also make a great lunchbox addition.

V DF **MAKES 20**   110 calories

A little rapeseed or olive oil, for greasing

130g dried, stoned prunes

130ml boiling water

Zest and juice of 1 orange

1 Cox's apple, cored and finely chopped

50g sultanas

100g jumbo or rolled oats

3 eggs

25g set honey

50g olive or rapeseed oil

50g spelt flour

50g wheatbran

1 tbsp baking powder

50g hazelnuts, roughly chopped

150g blackberries

- Preheat the oven to 190°C/375°F/Gas mark 5. Grease and line a 20cm square cake tin with baking parchment.

- Put the prunes into a bowl and pour over the boiling water. Set aside to soak. Mix the orange zest, juice, apple and sultanas together in a separate bowl.

- Put the oats into a mini food processor and whizz to make a fine flour.

- Drain the prunes, reserving the liquid, then whizz in a food processor until smooth. Stir the liquid back in, then spoon this mixture into a sieve resting over a bowl, and use a spoon to extract the purée. You should have 140–160g.

- Whisk the eggs, honey and oil in a bowl until foamy – this will take around 3 minutes, then fold in the prune purée, apple mixture, oats, oil, spelt flour, wheatbran, baking powder and hazelnuts. Fold everything together to combine.

- Spoon the mixture into the cake tin, then scatter over the blackberries. Bake in the oven for around 40 minutes, until a skewer inserted into the centre comes out clean. Cool on a wire rack, then cut into 20 squares and serve.

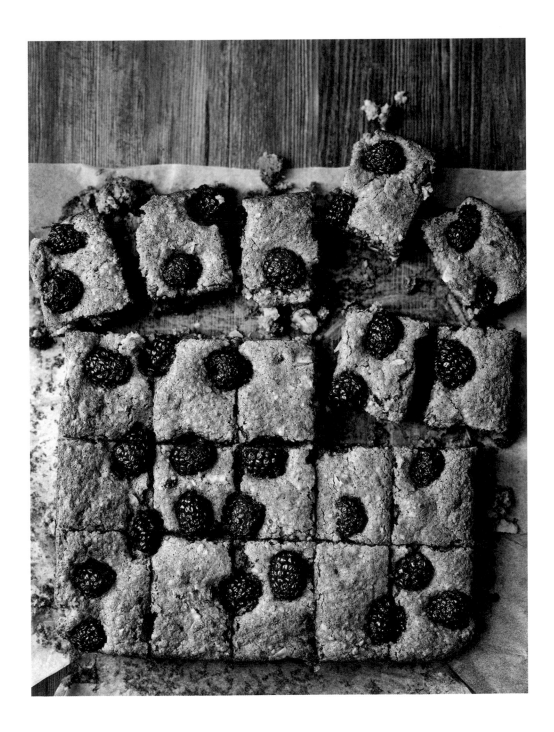

Sugar-free Cocoa-dusted Truffles

These are so good, I promise you, and make a wonderful little present to take along when visiting a friend. The dates should be the soft kind so they blend well with the other ingredients, and it is important to use both types of almonds – ground and whole – for their different textures.

 V DF GF MAKES 16 TRUFFLES   41 calories

40g ready-to-eat dried dates, roughly chopped

Zest of ¼ orange

50g dark chocolate (100% cocoa solids),
   roughly chopped

25g whole almonds, toasted

10g ground almonds

1 tbsp just-boiled water

1–2 tbsp cocoa powder

- Put the chopped dates in a mini food processor with the orange zest, dark chocolate and both types of almonds. Blend everything together to chop the ingredients finely, until the mixture looks crumbly.

- Add the boiled water and blend again to make a ganache. The heat of the water will just melt the chocolate enough to bring the mixture together.

- Spoon the ganache into a bowl and use a teaspoon to scoop up pieces about the size of a Malteser, and roll them into a ball. Do this until you have 16 balls.

- Sprinkle the cocoa powder on to a flat plate and toss the balls in it. Pop them in the fridge to firm up, but take them out 10–15 minutes before eating. Store in an airtight container for up to 1 week.

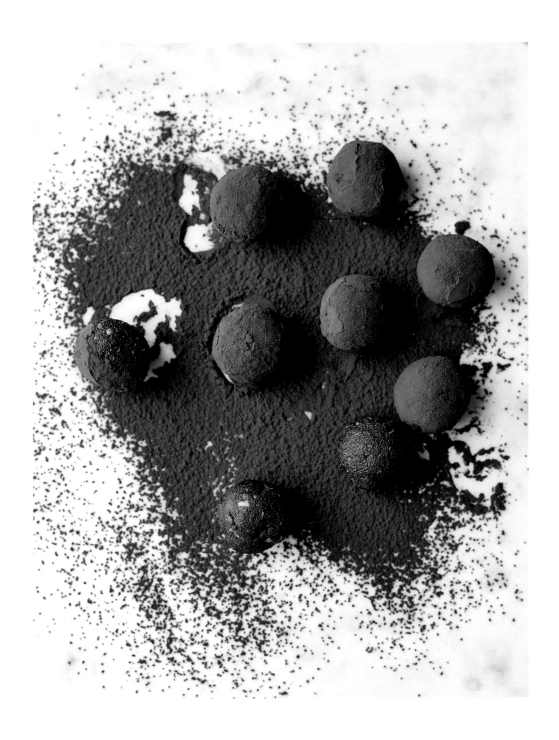

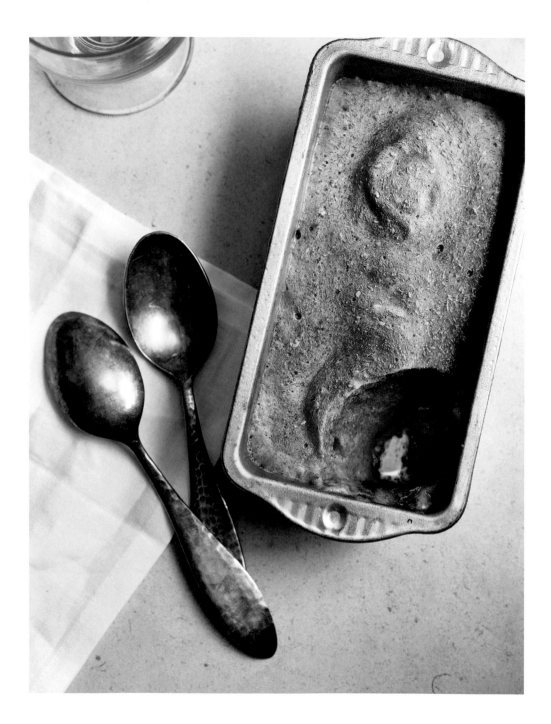

Quick Banana Ice Cream

No sugar, no cream – this is the quickest ever ice cream and perfectly healthy, too!

V DF GF **SERVES 4**   66 calories

250g peeled bananas   150g frozen raspberries

- Chop the bananas into pieces, put them on a plate, then put them in the freezer for 30–45 minutes, until the pieces are frozen but not completely hard.
- Put the frozen banana pieces in a food processor with the raspberries and blitz until the two ingredients blend together into an ice cream. If you like a soft-scoop texture to your ice cream, serve it like this.
- Otherwise, for a more set ice cream, transfer to a freezer-proof box and freeze for a further 10–20 minutes to firm up, then serve.

Banana Ice Lollies with Toasted Coconut

My family all love this sweet treat, which is such fun to make. If you freeze the bananas for about half an hour they'll be deliciously firm and chilled but not ice-cold or difficult to eat.

V DF GF SERVES 4   132 calories

2 bananas

50g dark chocolate (around 90% cocoa solids)

15g unsweetened desiccated coconut

Pinch cinnamon

- Cut each banana in half through the middle and, without peeling, push a wooden skewer or lolly stick into the cut end. Transfer them to the freezer and freeze for 30 minutes (use the fast-freeze compartment if you have one).

- Melt the chocolate in a bowl resting over a pan of boiling water, making sure the base doesn't touch the water. Set aside to cool a little. Alternatively, you can put the chocolate in a bowl and melt it in the microwave on low.

- Put the coconut into a frying pan with the cinnamon and toast for 2–3 minutes, until golden.

- Peel the banana and spoon or drizzle the chocolate over the end. Sprinkle the coconut over the top, and serve.

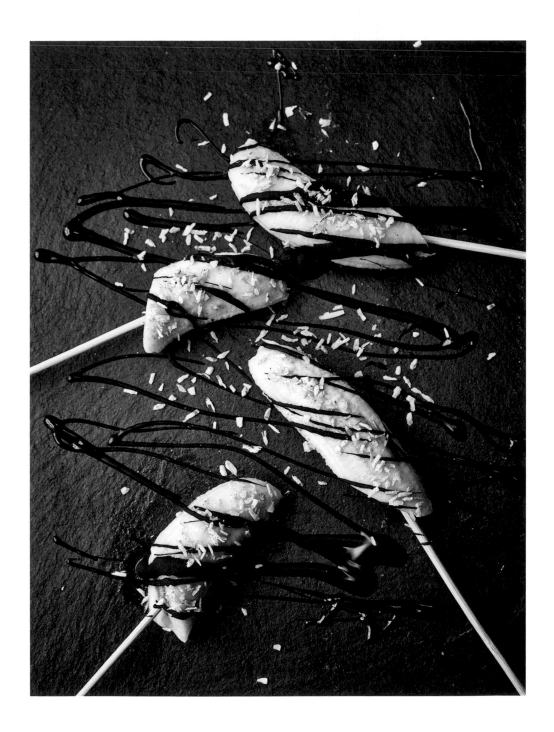

BREADS AND BASICS

Fruit and Nut Loaf

I've suggested using white or wholemeal spelt flour for this bread – both are good but the white flour makes a slightly lighter loaf. The nuts make it really nutritious and give it a lovely crunchy texture.

V DF   MAKES 1 LOAF/12 SLICES   161 calories per slice

10g dried yeast
½ tsp honey
250–275ml lukewarm water
250g wholemeal flour, plus extra for dusting
100g white or wholemeal spelt flour
50g dried apricots, finely chopped

25g hazelnuts, chopped
25g walnuts, chopped
20g flaked almonds
1 tsp finely ground sea salt
1 tbsp olive or rapeseed oil, plus extra for oiling

- Put the yeast and honey into a small bowl. Pour over about a third of the water, then stir the ingredients together. Set aside for 5–10 minutes to allow the yeast to activate.

- Sift the flours into a large bowl. Add the apricots, hazelnuts, walnuts, flaked almonds and salt. Stir everything together. Make a well in the middle and pour in the olive or rapeseed oil.

- Pour the yeast mixture into the middle, too, rinsing out the bowl with the remaining water to dissolve any bits of yeast if necessary, and pouring this into the bowl, too.

- Stir well with a round-bladed knife or wooden spoon to make a rough dough, then use your hands to bring everything together. It will be sticky, but resist adding any flour otherwise the finished loaf will be heavy. Put it on a board and knead for about 5 minutes, until soft and sticky. Put it in a clean bowl, cover and leave in a warm place for 40 minutes.

- Lightly oil a 500g loaf tin, then dust it heavily with flour. Take the dough out of the bowl and put it on a board. Shape it into an oval and push it into the loaf tin, easing it into the corners. Set aside again for about 30 minutes. Preheat the oven to the highest setting.

- Turn the oven down to 200°C/400°F/Gas mark 6 then put the loaf in the oven and bake for about 30 minutes. Ease it out of its tin, then turn it upside down and rest it on the top of the tin and return it to the oven for a further 15 minutes, until the bread is cooked. Check by taking the loaf out of the tin and lightly tapping the base – it's ready when it sounds hollow.

- Transfer the loaf to a wire rack to cool and serve with a slick of butter, or one of the nut butters and the low-sugar berry compote (see pages 121 and 231).

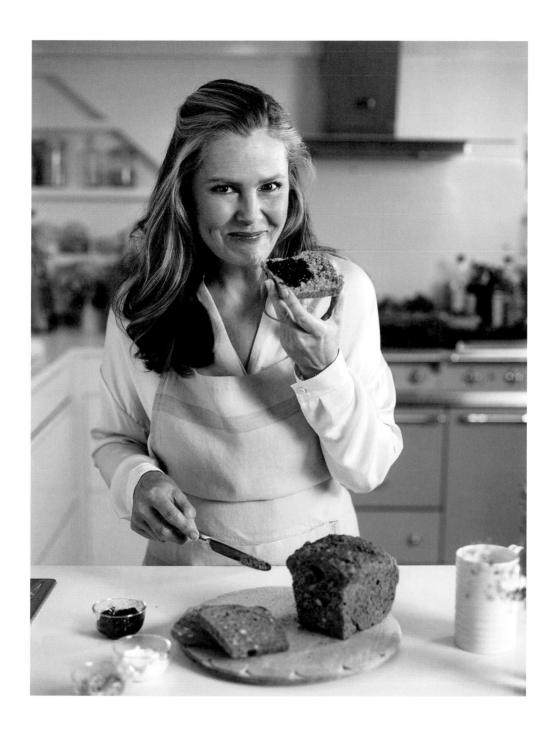

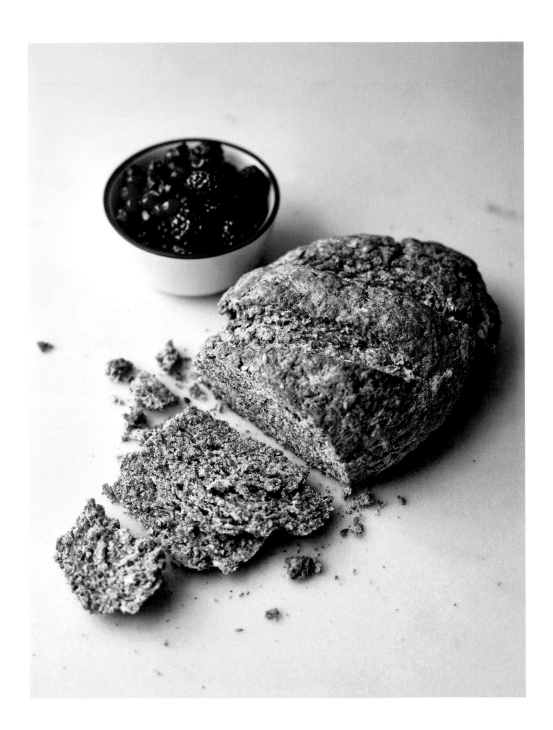

Rough and Tumble Bread

This dense little loaf of goodness is so called because you mix all the ingredients together roughly, tumble it all out of the bowl, then shape it and bake it. It doesn't contain any white flour, so it's very wholesome. Great served warm, with scrambled eggs.

v   SERVES 8   200 calories

A little olive oil, for greasing
100g wholemeal flour
100g spelt flour
50g jumbo or rolled oats
1 tbsp baking powder

2 tbsp linseeds
1 tsp sea salt
50g chilled unsalted butter
150ml whole milk

- Preheat the oven to 200°C/400°F/Gas mark 6. Lightly grease a non-stick baking sheet with a little oil. Put the wholemeal flour, spelt flour and oats into a large bowl. Add the baking powder, linseeds and salt, and mix everything together.

- Grate the butter straight into the bowl. Stir it into the dry mix with a table knife, chopping the strands up as you do this.

- Make a well in the middle and pour in the milk. Use the knife to mix everything again, then tip the mixture out on to a board. Shape it with your hands into an oval and mark a couple of times on top with the knife. Alternatively, roughly shape it into a round and mark into quarters.

- Transfer the dough to the baking sheet, sprinkle any leftover flour in the bowl over the top and bake for 30–35 minutes, until golden – and it should sound hollow when you tap the base. Cool on a wire rack, then serve.

LIZ'S TIP

To make a low-sugar berry compote, put 850g of thawed frozen mixed summer fruit and any juice into a saucepan with 50g of set honey. Use a sharp knife to scrape down the length of 1 vanilla pod to open it and release the seeds, then swap to a round-bladed table knife and run that down the middle to release the seeds. Put the seeds and the pod into the saucepan. Bring to the boil, then turn the heat down low and simmer for 20 minutes until syrupy, stirring every now and then to make sure it doesn't burn. Freeze for up to 1 month or keep for 4 days in the fridge in a sealable container.

Spelt Flatbreads

These are just right with the lamb kebabs on page 204 and also great served with some mustard and cheese dip and topped with shredded salad. You can also use this dough to make a bannock-style breakfast bread – see my tip below.

v MAKES 4   229 calories

200g spelt flour, plus extra for dusting   ½ tsp salt
1 tsp linseeds   100g Greek yoghurt
½ tbsp baking powder   75ml milk

- Sift the flour into a large, wide bowl. Stir in the seeds, baking powder and salt.

- Make a well in the middle and add the yoghurt and milk. Use a table knife to mix them first, then continue to stir to bring the mixture together. Knead lightly in the bowl, mopping up all the excess flour until you have a soft, smooth dough. Divide the dough into four.

- Dust a board lightly with a little flour, then dust the rolling pin, too. Roll out one piece of dough until you have a round that measures 18–19cm. It should be very thin.

- Heat a large frying pan over a medium heat until hot, and put the rolled-out round into the pan. Cook for 1–2 minutes until bubbles start to appear on top, then turn over and cook the other side for a further minute, until golden.

- Continue to roll and cook each piece of dough to make four flatbreads.

LIZ'S TIP

For a bannock-style bread for breakfast, which is slightly smaller in size but thicker and great for spreading with a little nut butter, do this: follow the recipe up to the end of the second step. When rolling out the dough, roll until it measures 13–14cm, shaping it into a round as you go. The dough will be about 5mm thick. Cook as above, but for 3 minutes on each side. You'll notice the round puffs up, and it'll look as though the top is drying out. Flip over and cook for a further 3 minutes, until golden underneath.

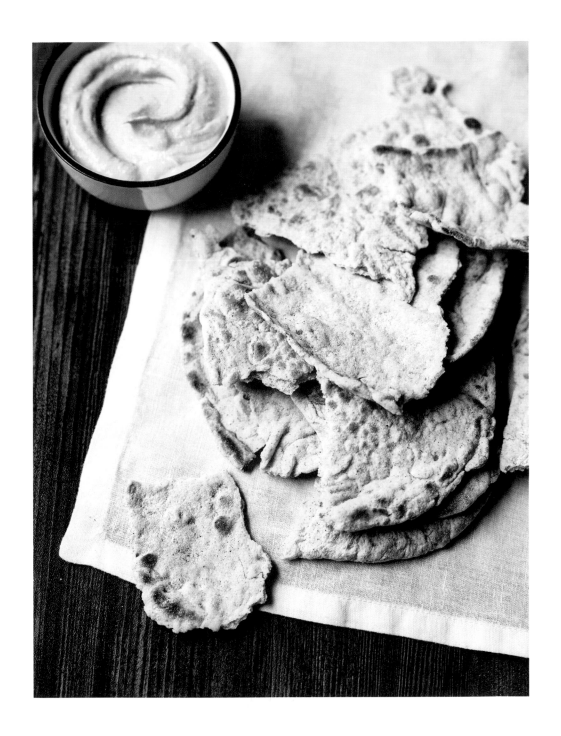

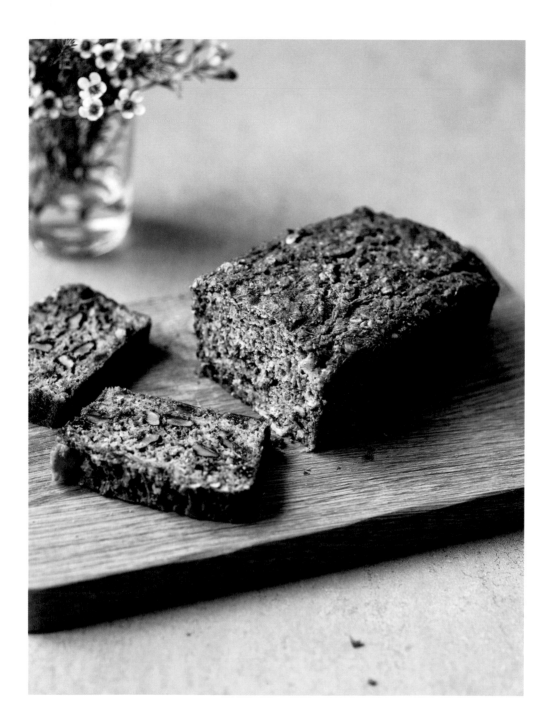

Courgette, Sultana and Walnut Loaf

Lots of good things in this loaf, which is great for breakfast with a poached egg or at teatime with some fruit compote (see page 231).

v   MAKES 1 LOAF/12 SLICES   100 Calories

150g courgette, grated
1 tsp lemon thyme leaves
½ tsp salt
40g sultanas
25g walnuts, chopped
125g spelt or wholemeal flour

25g oats
50g Cheddar cheese, grated
2 tsp baking powder
100ml milk
1 egg, beaten

- Preheat the oven to 180°C/350°F/Gas mark 4. Put a loaf tin liner into a 450g loaf tin and set aside.

- Put the courgette, lemon thyme, salt, sultanas and walnuts into a bowl and mix everything together. Add the flour, oats, cheese and baking powder and mix again.

- Whisk together the milk and egg, then make a well in the middle of the courgette mixture and pour it in. Fold everything together. Spoon the mixture into the tin and bake for 1 hour 15 minutes to 1 hour 30 minutes, or until a skewer comes out clean. Take the loaf out of the tin and cool on a wire rack.

Basil Dressing

This is lovely used as soon as it's made but will also keep well in the fridge for up to 5 days, stored in an airtight container. The oil solidifies so it also makes a great spread, slathered on toasted rye and topped with scrambled eggs for breakfast.

V DF GF   MAKES 8 SERVINGS   50 calories

15g basil leaves and stalks	½ garlic clove, crushed
10g pine nuts	Sea salt and freshly
50ml olive oil	ground black pepper

• Put the basil, pine nuts, olive oil and garlic into a food processor. Blend until smooth. Season well, then whizz again. Taste to check the seasoning and adjust accordingly.

Pumpkin Seed Dressing

I use this dressing all the time – it's one of my very favourites. Pumpkin seeds are rich in antioxidants and magnesium and so are a valuable food.

V DF GF   MAKES 4 SERVINGS   140 calories

25g pumpkin seeds	½ shallot, finely chopped
4 tbsp olive oil	1 tbsp white wine vinegar
2 gem lettuce leaves	Sea salt and freshly ground black pepper
1 tbsp chopped fresh dill	
1 tbsp chopped fresh chives	

• Put all the ingredients into a food processor, and season well. Add 2 tablespoons of cold water and whizz until smooth. You may need to stop the processor halfway through and scrape down the ingredients to make sure they're all finely chopped.

Apple Cider Vinaigrette

I'm a big fan of organic apple cider vinegar and I like to use it in this tangy vinaigrette.

V DF GF MAKES 10 SERVINGS   81 calories

4 tbsp extra virgin olive oil
4 tbsp flaxseed oil
5 tbsp cider vinegar
½ tsp mustard powder
½ tsp mustard seeds
1 tsp fresh thyme leaves
Salt and freshly ground black pepper

- Put all the ingredients into a jar, and season well. Seal and shake until the mixture emulsifies. Add 1 teaspoon of water to help it on its way if necessary. Store in the fridge for up to 2 weeks.

Mustard Dressing

The hit of Dijon mustard makes this a really flavoursome dressing to wake up a red cabbage slaw or other salad.

V DF GF MAKES 8 SERVINGS   56 calories

1 tbsp Dijon mustard
10g rocket
2 tbsp extra virgin olive oil
2 tbsp rapeseed oil
1 tsp red wine vinegar
1 tsp mustard seeds
Sea salt and freshly ground black pepper

- Put the mustard, rocket, oils and vinegar into a mini food processor and whizz to chop up the rocket and make a dressing. Add 1 teaspoon of water and season well, then whizz again to blend, scraping down the sides to ensure that all the bits are incorporated. Taste again to check the seasoning.

- Spoon the dressing into a small jar and add the mustard seeds, then give everything another good shake. Store in the fridge for up to 5 days.

Vegetable Stock

This is the easiest of all the stocks as you can just use whatever vegetables you have to hand. I've suggested a selection below. Don't add salt – just season whatever dish you're making with the stock.

V DF GF MAKES 12 CUBES   3 calories

2 unpeeled shallots, halved	1 bay leaf
1 celery stick, halved	1 sprig rosemary
1 carrot, quartered	1 sprig thyme
1 broccoli stalk, quartered	6 black peppercorns

- Put all the ingredients into a pan and pour over 1 litre of cold water. Cover with a lid and bring to the boil.

- Turn the heat down very low and simmer for 1 hour. Strain the contents of the pan through a sieve and into a clean pan.

- Put the pan back on the heat and bring to the boil, then cook until the liquid has reduced to around 180ml.

- Cool, then divide between a standard 12-hole ice-cube tray. Freeze and use within 1 month. To use, pop a cube of frozen stock into a jug and pour over 250ml of hot water.

Chicken Stock

I love having my own chicken stock cubes in the freezer to use at a moment's notice. I don't add salt to the stock, as I prefer to season the dish I'm making.

DF GF MAKES 12 CUBES   10 calories

1 fresh chicken carcass (or use a stripped one, left over from a Sunday roast or from Roast Lemon Chicken with Spring Vegetables, page 196)	1 onion, halved
	1 carrot, cut into 3 pieces
	1 celery stick, halved
	2 bay leaves
	1 sprig rosemary
	2–3 sprigs thyme
	8 black peppercorns

- Put the chicken carcass into a large saucepan and add the remaining ingredients. Cover with cold water, then put a lid on the pan and bring to the boil. Skim off any scum floating on the surface.

- Turn the heat down to a very low simmer and cook for about 1 hour. After about half an hour, the liquid will have reduced, so turn the carcass over to cook the exposed part, too.

- Strain into a clean pan. Bring the liquid to the boil and reduce until the liquid measures around 180ml. Pour the liquid into a 12-hole ice cube tray and freeze. Use within 1 month. To use, pop a cube of frozen stock into a jug and pour over 250ml of hot water.

Beef Stock

If you don't want to put the oven on specially for this you can roast the bones under a Sunday joint instead.

DF **GF** MAKES 12 CUBES   8 calories

1kg beef bones
1 carrot, halved
1 celery stick, halved
1 onion, halved, or use 4 whole unpeeled shallots

1 tbsp olive or rapeseed oil
6 black peppercorns
2 bay leaves
1 sprig thyme

- Preheat the oven to 200°C/400°F/Gas mark 6. Spread the beef bones out in a large flameproof roasting tin. Add the carrot, celery and onion, and drizzle with the oil.

- Pour 150ml of cold water into the tin, then transfer to the oven and roast for 45 minutes to 1 hour, until all the bones have browned. Transfer the bones to a large saucepan. Drain any fat away from the tin, then pour in enough water to cover the base. Heat on the hob, stirring well, to dissolve all the brown juices from the pan into the water.

- Pour the liquid into the pan, then add the peppercorns, bay and thyme. Cover and bring to the boil. Skim off any scum and discard, then turn the heat down and simmer for 1 hour. Strain the liquid into a clean pan and bring to the boil. Simmer until the liquid has reduced to about 180ml, then cool and pour into a standard 12-hole ice-cube tray. To use, pop a cube of frozen stock into a jug and pour over 250ml of hot water.

Fish Stock

Your fishmonger will gladly provide you with fish trimmings for making stock and it's no trouble to do. The bay leaves will fill your kitchen with a wonderfully aromatic scent as the stock bubbles away.

DF **GF** MAKES 12 CUBES   4 calories

2 skeletons of fish, including the heads, such as sea bass
1 shallot, chopped

1 celery stick, chopped
2 bay leaves
8 black peppercorns

- Put all the ingredients into a large saucepan. Cover with 1.8 litres of cold water and put a lid on the pan. Bring to the boil, then turn the heat down low and simmer for 30 minutes.

- Strain, then returnthe liquid to the pan and simmer, uncovered, until the liquid has reduced to around 180ml.

- Cool, then divide between a standard 12-hole ice-cube tray. Freeze and use within 1 month. To use, pop a cube of frozen stock into a jug and pour over 250ml of hot water.

DRINKS AND SMOOTHIES

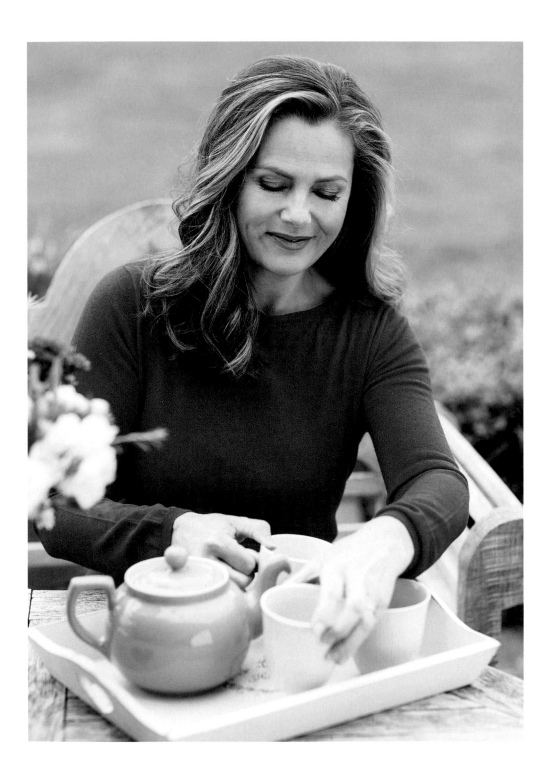

Lemongrass, Ginger and Mint Tea

This fresh and uplifting cleansing cuppa is a perfect internal skin soother. The antimicrobial and antibacterial properties of lemongrass and ginger work well with fresh mint leaves – which are packed with antioxidants to help to reduce skin inflammation, too.

V DF GF SERVES 1   7 calories

2 lemongrass stalks
1 thumb-sized piece fresh root ginger,
    peeled and roughly chopped

10 fresh mint leaves
Freshly boiled water

Cut off the ends of the lemongrass and remove any dry outer leaves. Bruise the lemongrass in a pestle and mortar (a heavy rolling pin on a chopping board will also work), then cut the stalks in half so they fit in a mug. Put the ginger into the mug, along with the mint leaves. Pour the boiling water over the lemongrass stalks, ginger and mint leaves and leave it to steep for 3–4 minutes before drinking (or make in a pot and refresh with hot water throughout the day).

Turmeric Tonic Tea

If you're in need of an afternoon pick-me-up, this refreshing and cleansing tea is just the thing – with an abundance of health benefits. Turmeric has long been used in traditional Indian medicine and skincare for its rejuvenating and anti-inflammatory properties, while ginger is rich in antibacterial compounds.

V DF GF SERVES 1   31 calories

1 tsp turmeric powder
1 thumb-sized piece fresh root ginger,
    peeled and roughly chopped
¼ lemon

1 tsp honey
Note: Manuka honey works particularly well
    here due to its additional anti-inflammatory and
    antibacterial properties.

Put the turmeric into a mug with the ginger. Squeeze the lemon quarter into the mug, and then drop it in. Pour over boiling water and then stir in the honey. Let it steep for a few minutes before drinking.

Lavender, Rosemary and Lemon Tea

Fragrant and aromatic, this botanical brew is full of skin-boosting properties – from the soothing lavender to the anti-inflammatory rosemary. The lemon gives it a refreshing kick.

V DF GF   SERVES 1   2 calories

2 sprigs lavender
3 sprigs rosemary

½ lemon
Freshly boiled water

Put the lavender and rosemary into a mug and then squeeze in the juice of the lemon half, before dropping it in. Pour over freshly boiled water and steep for 3 minutes or so before enjoying.

Rosebud and Cardamom Tea

This Middle Eastern-inspired fusion of floral rosebuds and aromatic cardamom pods makes a deliciously fragrant skin-friendly tea. Rosebuds have long been associated with promoting health and beauty, due to their vitamin C content, while cardamom pods are bursting with magnesium and antioxidants to help keep skin youthfully glowing.

V DF GF   SERVES 1   2 calories

1 tsp cardamon pods
2 tsp dried rosebuds
Hot water

Note: Dried rose petals also work well, but avoid using shop-bought roses which may have been sprayed with pesticides.

In a pestle and mortar, crush up the cardamom pods to release their flavour then put them into a mug, followed by the rosebuds. Pour over water that has almost been brought up to the boil, and let it steep for approximately 3 minutes. If you prefer a clear liquid, strain out the rosebuds and cardamom pods with a tea strainer.

Blueberry, Pear and Yoghurt Smoothie

The perfect way to start the day, this feel-good smoothie is full of skin-nourishing goodness. Blueberries are packed full of antioxidants, while the fibre-rich pear contains collagen-boosting vitamin C to help skin stay firm and radiant. The beneficial probiotic bacteria found in live yoghurt also help keep skin smooth and clear.

V GF SERVES 1   370 calories

2 pears, cored and roughly chopped   200ml natural live yoghurt
150g blueberries   ¼ lemon
                                            splash of organic milk or almond milk (optional)

Put the pears in a blender with the blueberries and yoghurt. Blend the ingredients well, then add in a squeeze of lemon. If you prefer your smoothie slightly thinner, add a splash of organic milk or almond milk. Stir well before serving.

Blackberry, Apple, Almond and Yoghurt Smoothie

Not only is this smoothie delicious, it's also bursting with skin-friendly nutrients. The antioxidant anthocyanins from the dark-skinned blackberries help guard against premature skin ageing, while the vitamin E, essential fatty acids and protein in the almond milk promote radiance.

V GF SERVES 1   308 calories

100g blackberries   100ml natural yoghurt
2 apples, cored and roughly chopped   Honey, to taste (optional)
150ml almond milk

Put the blackberries, apples, almond milk and natural yoghurt into a blender or food processor and blend until smooth. Add honey to taste, if using.

NOTE: Use pure almond milk made with just almonds and water (or make your own).

Beetroot, Carrot and Apple Juice with Ginger

This vibrant and energising juice will not only put a spring in your step but is also full of skin-enhancing vitamins and minerals. Both beetroot and carrot are especially rich in beta-carotene and vitamin C – key players in promoting a clear and glowing complexion. Truly a classic skin-friendly combo.

V DF GF SERVES 1   83 calories

2 medium beetroots, scrubbed and tops trimmed   1 green apple, cored
2 carrots   1 thumb-sized piece fresh root ginger

Juice all the ingredients together. Mix together well before serving.

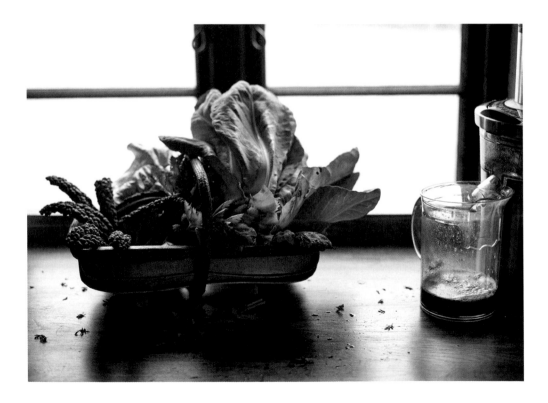

Resources and Suppliers

THE FOLLOWING ARE RELIABLE RESOURCES
OF INFORMATION

Liz Earle Wellbeing
The home of Liz's latest research, wellbeing wisdom and more.

Sign up to receive free newsletters, details of special offers and events to meet Liz.
lizearlewellbeing.com

Cosmetic Toiletry and Perfumery Association
CTPA.org

Consumer information
thefactsabout.co.uk

European product safety and legislation
ec.europa.eu/growth/sectors/cosmetics

European community
cosmeticseurope.eu

US-based skincare and cosmetics information
personalcarecouncil.org

SUPPLIERS

SKINCARE

Liz Earle Beauty Co.
Official website and online sales for the Liz Earle beauty brand
www.lizearle.com

ESSENTIAL OILS, HERBS AND SUPPLEMENTS

Baldwins Natural Herbs
One of the UK's leading, longest running herbal supplier
baldwins.co.uk

Efamol
The leading suppliers of genuine Rigel seed evening primrose oil supplements for help with eczema and skin health
efamol.com

Manuka honey
Reputable website selling genuine UMF-rated Manuka honey
manukahoney.co.uk

Naturya
Purveyors of high quality, nutrient-rich superfoods and powders
naturya.com

Probiotics

Two of my favourite formulae are Dr Mercola's Complete Probiotics supplement and Sweet Cures Probiotic Blend. Both companies have informative websites.

mercola.com

sweet-cures.com

Pukka

Excellent on-line resource and shop for herbal products, notably skin health herbs

Pukkaherbs.com

Tisserand

One of the best UK suppliers of pure essential oils

tisserand.com

WATER FILTERS AND FILTER BOTTLES

Brita

The leading brand for water filters including jug filters, under-sink filters, water-filter kettles and portable filter water bottles

brita.co.uk

Bobble

Portable water bottles and filters

waterbobble.com

The National Eczema Society

National Eczema Society
11 Murray Street
London NW19RE
www.eczema.org

The National Institute of Medical Herbalists

Clover House
James Court
South Street
Exeter EX1 1EE
Telephone 01392 426022
E-mail: info@nimh.org.uk
http://www.nimh.org.uk

Chelsea Physic Garden

Dating back to 1673, the garden is a tranquil oasis in central London and home to over 5000 living medicinal and therapeutic plants.

chelseaphysicgarden.co.uk

Reflexology

Association of Reflexologists
Discover more information and find your nearest UK therapist AoR.org.uk

Acknowledgements

I am grateful to many talented people who have helped to make this beautiful book happen. Firstly, to my literary agent Rosemary Sandberg for bringing me together with Amanda Harris at Orion. I am so thankful for Amanda giving me the opportunity to launch a brand new imprint with her at Orion Spring. I'm looking forward to creating many more brilliant books together! Also to her talented team, including Helen Ewing, Jillian Young and Liz Jones, and especially my editor Jinny Johnson, who I have loved working so closely with. I'm also grateful to leading dietitian Fiona Hunter for her professional expertise. A heartfelt thank you to Emma Marsden who worked with me on many of the oh-so delicious and nutritious recipes, and to Polly Beard and my entire Liz Earle Wellbeing team who helped in my Wellbeing Studios with research, testing and tasting… We've had such a great time working on all this together.

A huge thank you to the brilliant Dan Jones and Lorenzo Mazzega for their gorgeous photographs, not just of me and my 'girls' Lily, Patricia and Indigo, but also for Dan's fabulous food photography. As well as thanks to home economist and food stylist Natalie Thomson, photography assistant Sophie Fox and to Caroline Clark for putting everything together in such a stylishly designed book. A special word of thanks to my make-up artist Kerry September and hair stylist Jonothon Malone, as well as to Lily Earle for co-ordinating wardrobe and accessories. This beautiful book is truly a result of fantastic teamwork and I am so grateful to you all and many more besides.

Liz x

Wellbeing Studios, London

WARDROBE CREDITS:

Cover: blue top, Brora
Inside cover: peach shirt, Jaeger
Pages 6 and 229: white shirt, The White Company; apron, The Linen Works
Pages 12 and 33: grey top, Jigsaw; linen apron, The Linen Works
Page 23: orange jumper, Brora; trousers The White Company; scarf, The Travel Wrap Company
Pages 26-27: white shirt, The White Company
Page 29: orange jumper, Brora; jeans, Hobbs,; gilet, Musto

Page 54: navy top, Jaeger
Page 57: orange top, Brora
Page 69: cream dressing gown, Liberty
Page 79: orange jumper, Brora; jeans, Hobbs; jacket, Barbour; scarf, The Travel Wrap Company; boots, Musto
Page 87: lilac wrap, Joseph
Page 140, navy top Jaeger
Page 182, blue jumper, Marks and Spencer, apron, The Linen Works

OVEN TEMPERATURE GUIDE

	Elec °C	Elec °F	Elec °C (Fan)	Gas mark
Very cool	110	225	90	¼
	120	250	100	½
Cool	140	275	120	1
	150	300	130	2
Moderate	160	325	140	3
	170	350	160	4
Moderately hot	190	375	170	5
	200	400	180	6
Hot	220	425	200	7
	230	450	210	8
Very hot	240	475	220	9

LIQUID MEASUREMENTS

Metric	Imperial	Australian/US
25ml	1 fl oz	
60ml	2 fl oz	¼ cup
75ml	3 fl oz	
100ml	3½ fl oz	
120ml	4 fl oz	½ cup
150ml	5 fl oz	
180ml	6 fl oz	¾ cup
200ml	7 fl oz	
250ml	9 fl oz	1 cup
300ml	10½ fl oz	1¼ cups
350ml	12½ fl oz	1½ cups
400ml	14 fl oz	1¾ cups
450ml	16 fl oz	2 cups
600ml	1 pint	2½ cups
750ml	1¼ pints	3 cups
900ml	1½ pints	3½ cups
1 litre	1¾ pints	1 quart or 4 cups
1.2 litres	2 pints	
1.4 litres	2½ pints	
1.5 litres	2¾ pints	
1.7 litres	3 pints	
2 litres	3½ pints	

WEIGHT MEASUREMENTS

Metric	Imperial
10g	½ oz
20g	¾ oz
25g	1 oz
40g	1½ oz
50g	2 oz
60g	2½ oz
75g	3 oz
110g	4 oz
125g	4½ oz
150g	5 oz
175g	6 oz
200g	7 oz
225g	8 oz
250g	9 oz
275g	10 oz
350g	12 oz
450g	1 lb
700g	1½ lb
900g	2 lb

Index

a

acid/alkaline foods 36–7
acne 15
advanced glycation end products (AGEs) 15
aerobic exercise 78
alcohol 18
alkaline greenie glow juice 38
alkaline skin smoothie 38
almond milk, home-made 97
anti-acne diet 45–6
anti-cellulite hip and thigh oil blend 59
anti-inflammatories 39
argan oil 52
aroma bath/shower 69
artichokes 30, 32, 33
artificial sweeteners 15
asparagus 30, 32
avocado oil 52, 55

b

barley grass 84
bath oil blends 71
bathroom cupboards detox 14–15
bitter leaves 30, 32
body brushing 16–17
body cleansing 28
body massage 59
body scrub 19
borage oil 52
breathing 67–8

c

cacay oil 52
caffeine 17, 26, 65
calming foods 36–8
camomile and rose herbal steam 35
canola (rapeseed) oil 55
carrot juice 32
chicory 30, 32
chlorella 48, 84
chocolate 16
cleansing routines 86
coconut oil 55
collagen 48

d

dandelions 30, 32
day creams 51
diet
    anti-acne 45–6
    low-GL 45–6
    plant oils in 53–5
    two-day detox 21–2
    dry-skin body brushing 16–17

e

eczema 28, 39
Epsom salts bath 47
essential fatty acids (EFAs) 39, 48
essential oils 69–71
eye creams 51
eyes 66–7

f

face masks 44
face scrub 19
facial cleansing 24–5
facial exercises 77
facial massage 56–7
facial oils 51
facial serums 51, 76
facials 83
fats: good fats 41–2
flaxseed oil 55
food combining diet 72
food cupboards detox 12–13
foot massage 73–4
foot scrub 62
fridge detox 12–13
fruits 41

g

ginger 17–18
globe artichokes 30, 32, 33
glycaemic load (GL) table 46
glycation 15
grains 42

h

hair 80–1
hair mask 81
hand scrub 63
healing skin drink 40
hemp seeds 84
herbal baths 47
herbal steams 34–5
herbal teas 17
herbs 84
hydration 18, 26–7

i

International Nomenclature of Cosmetic Ingredients (INCI) 14

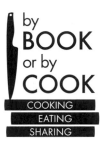

For more delicious recipes, features, videos and exclusives from Orion's cookery writers, and to sign up for our 'Recipe of the Week' email visit **bybookorbycook.co.uk**

Follow us

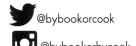 @bybookorcook

@bybookorbycook

Find us

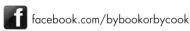 facebook.com/bybookorbycook

About Liz

Liz Earle MBE is one of Britain's most respected and trusted authorities on beauty and wellbeing. The award-winning author of over 30 best-selling books on nutrition, diet, skincare and natural health, she co-founded the eponymous global beauty brand Liz Earle Beauty Co. in 1995, before moving back to writing and broadcasting, now publishing the leading quarterly magazine *Liz Earle Wellbeing*.

An expert in feel-good-food and eating well for better beauty, her straightforward, balanced approach is trusted by millions of women worldwide. With a passion for demystifying science and de-bunking beauty myths, Liz's measured voice of reason has a deservedly large and loyal following in print, digital, on TV and online.

Travelling the globe for research, Liz comes home to roost on an organic farm in the UK's West Country with her husband and five children.

www.lizearlewellbeing.com

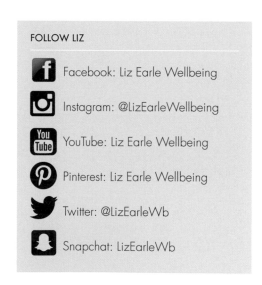

FOLLOW LIZ

Facebook: Liz Earle Wellbeing

Instagram: @LizEarleWellbeing

YouTube: Liz Earle Wellbeing

Pinterest: Liz Earle Wellbeing

Twitter: @LizEarleWb

Snapchat: LizEarleWb